AF364243

Application of Spectral Studies in Pharmaceutical Product Development

(Basic Approach with Illustrated Examples)

Application of Spectral Studies in Pharmaceutical Product Development

(Basic Approach with Illustrated Examples)

Dr. Ramalingam Peraman

Dr. Y. Padmanabha Reddy

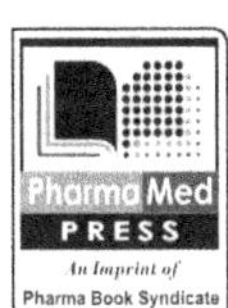

PharmaMed Press

An imprint of Pharma Book Syndicate

A unit of BSP Books Pvt. Ltd.

4-4-309/316, Giriraj Lane,

Sultan Bazar, Hyderabad - 500 095.

Application of Spectral Studies in Pharmaceutical Product Development (Basic Approach with Illustrated Examples) *by Ramalingam Peraman and Y. Padmanabha Reddy*

Published by

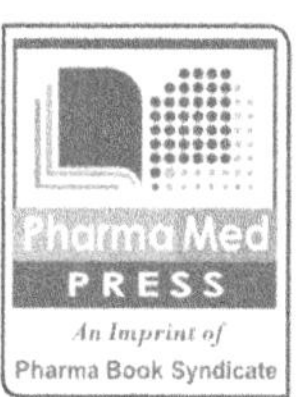

PharmaMed Press

An imprint of Pharma Book Syndicate

A unit of BSP Books Pvt. Ltd.

4-4-309/316, Giriraj Lane, Sultan Bazar, Hyderabad - 500 095.

Phone: 040-23445600, 23445688; Fax: 91+40-23445611

e-mail: info@pharmamedpress.com

www.pharmamedpress.com/pharmamedpress.net

ISBN: 978-93-88305-96-9

FOREWORD

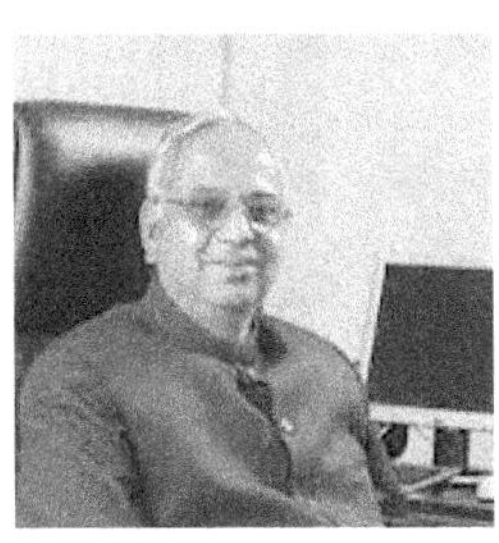

Prof. C. K. Kokate
M. Pharm., PhD

I am delighted to know that Dr. P. Ramalingam and Dr. Y. Padmanabha Reddy have jointly made their effort to bring out this book entitled "Application of Spectral studies in Pharmaceutical Product development (Basic Approach with Illustrated Examples)". I am extremely happy to write foreword, because the book is the first of its kind where the authors emphasized to compile various applications of spectral studies in pharmaceutical research.

I am amazed to see the explanations are illustrated with pharmaceutical products and absolutely filled with updated applications of Spectral studies including UV, IR, Raman, NMR, ESR and Mass spectroscopic techniques. In addition, authors have also added principle and instrumentation of few recent sophisticated techniques such as LC-MS/MS, LC-NMR, q-NMR, SEM/TEM etc.

I feel this book should be a better choice for young researchers, PG and UG students belonging to the disciplines of pharmaceutical, life and chemical sciences.

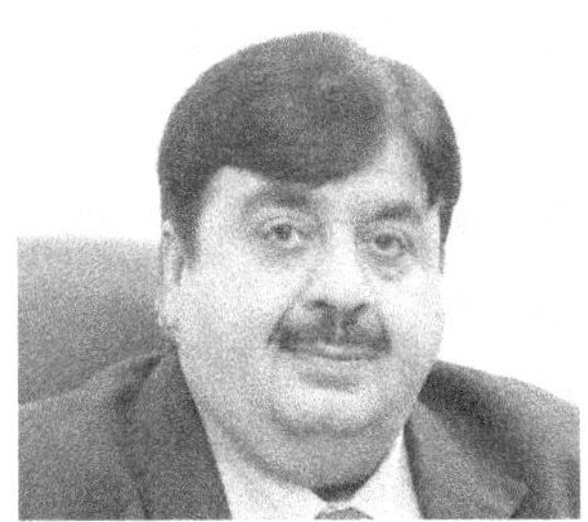

Dr. B. Suresh
M. Pharm.. PhD

The Book titled *""Application of Spectral Studies in Pharmaceutical Product Development (Basic approach with illustrated examples)"* brought out jointly by Dr. P. Ramalingam and Dr. Y. Padmanabha Reddy, is compiled several chapters under suitable headings, keeping in view of development of pharmaceuticals which brought the revolution in human health. In view of pharmaceutical development, the analytical techniques are serving as quality indicators throughout the life cycle of the drugs. The goal of this book is rightly pointed by authors to apply the spectral and result data with illustrated examples to various analytical techniques in the assessment of product formation and characterization using SEM/TEM, LC-MS/MS and LC-NMR.

I am glad that authors have made every attempt to create a document which meets all the needs of application and is different approach of presentation which will help all learners including researchers from industry and academia.

PREFACE

With our teaching and research experience to pharmacy graduates, it is our opinion that majority of graduates acquire adequate knowledge on principle and instrumentation component of analytical methods. But there are declined skills among budding graduate and young researchers on application aspects of spectral and advanced analytical data during real time product development.

Hence, we have taken tremendous effort to compile this book with a special emphasis on basics and interpretation of analytical results of various pharmaceutically important experimental techniques in development of pharmaceuticals. We strongly believe that learning the concept on examples will definitely enhance the knowledge and skills of the graduates. Hence, we have compiled the text book with lot of illustrated examples of spectra for various spectral techniques and few advanced techniques of pharmaceutical industries including LC-MS/MS, LC-NMR, q-NMR, SEM/TEM etc.

We are very much enthusiastic of this book which is new approach for the first time on learning of spectral interpretation and should be a better choice for young researchers, PG and UG students belonging to the disciplines of pharmaceutical, life and chemical sciences.

We also appreciate the publishers for the wonderful effort in bring out the new dimension of spectral interpretation.

Dr. P. Ramalingam

Dr. Y. Padmanabha Reddy

CONTENTS

Chapter 1

UV-Visible Spectroscopy

Spectroscopy and **spectrography** are the techniques based on the measurement of radiation intensity (absorbed or emitted or scattered by the sample or analyte) as a function of wavelength. Spectral measurement instruments are more commonly referred as spectrometers, spectrophotometers, spectrographs or spectral analyzers. These instruments measure the light intensity or resultant light from sample, (emitted or transmitted or scattered). Absorption is the measure of difference between incident and transmitted light (Figure 1.1).

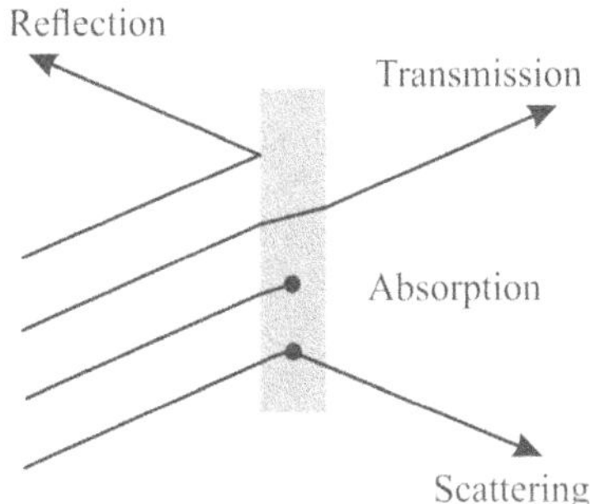

Figure 1.1 Various interaction of effect of light with matter (Analyte).

The output of scan measurement of sample from a range of wavelength is represented as 2D or 3D spectrum. In general X axis (Input) will be wavelength, Y axis (output) will be light absorbed (UV-Visible, IR, NMR or any absorption spectroscopy, Light emitted (fluorescence or any emission spectroscopy) or scattered (intensity of scatted light Raman spectroscopy). There are three types of Spectrum produced by spectroscopy

1. Continuous spectrum
2. Emission lines
3. Absorption lines

Selection Region based on Sample Nature

The difference between UV and Visible spectroscopy is the wavelength region used in measurement. UV region (190-380 nm) for colorless sample and visible region 380-790 nm for coloured sample. As result of scanning of sample using the light, the spectrum obtained is characteristic of sample / molecule nature, its highly depends on double bonds (pi electrons) configuration of the structure.

Absorption/Emission of Light by a Chemical Molecule

The mechanism behind the absorption of light by a molecule (analyte) or / and emission of light from the molecule (Analyte) is depends on the phenomena of electronic excitation / transition (Figure 1.2). The amount (probability) or type of the electron (sigma, pi, n) involved in the excitation determine the characteristic photon energy absorbed or emitted, will determine the shape and pattern of UV-Visible Spectrum.

As no two chemical molecules will have same number of electrons or configuration, the UV spectrum will be different for different compounds.

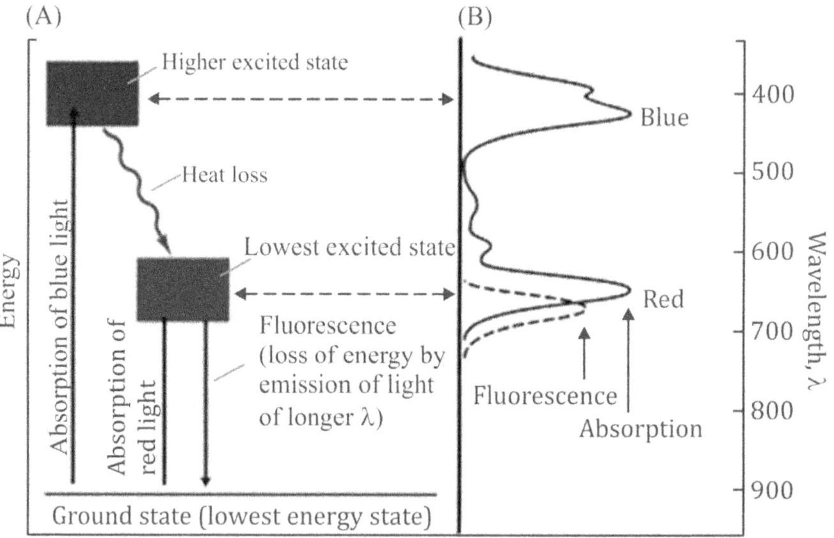

Figure 1.2 Absorption and emission process of matter (Analyte).

- The above figure shows the electronic excitation process and relaxation process of electron of molecule when UV-Visible light is irradiated on sample.

- Blue light and red light is indicated to understand the wavelength comparison.
- *NOTE*: sample should be low concentration, pure and highly transparent for any qualitative and quantitative analysis

Types of Electronic Transitions

- There are different types of electronic transition take place in the molecule, and each molecule undergoes more than one electronic transition, and requires different energy (Figure 1.3).
- Sigma transitions are higher takes in very low wavelength of UV region or in Vacuum UV region (< 190 nm).
- The below diagram indicate the comparison of different electronic transition and energy in which n' electron transition require less energy (absorbs higher wavelength)

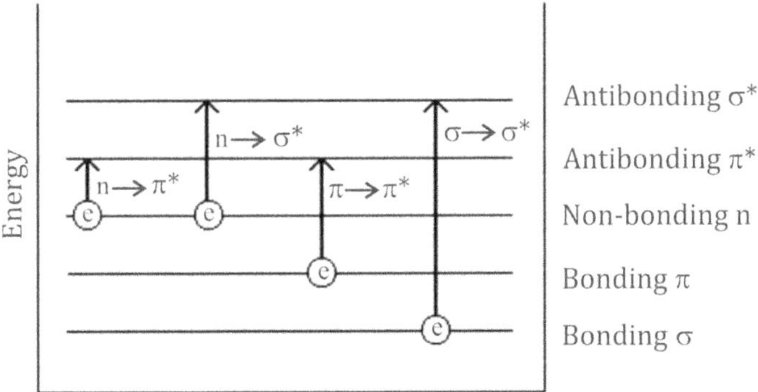

Figure 1.3 Types of electronic transition in a organic molecules upon UV-Visible light exposure.

From above figure, we can observe that the energy required for sigma transition (alkane) is the highest which is not available in UV region, so sigma transition may not be a practically observed. sigma transition may be possible at vacuum UV region (<190 nm).

How to predict the possible electronic transition for the given structure?

To predict the possible transition, we need to know the chemical structure and type of electrons available.

Table 1.1 Transition and Chemical structures

Chemical class	Types electron	Possible transitions (theoretical)
Alkane	Sigma electron only	Sigma to sigma*
Alkene (C=C), Benzene, Alkynes	Sigma and Pi electrons	Sigma to sigma* Pi to Pi*
Aldehyde, ketones, heterocyclic, acids, esters, (all compounds containing C=O, C=S	Sigma, pi electrons n' electrons	All type of transitions
Complexes	n' electrons	Charge transfer mechanism

Schematic Procedure in Measuring Absorbance

- In the instrumentation, always a monochromatic light will be used to measure an absorbance (in quantitative analysis).

- The monochromatic light to be used has to be selected from the UV spectrum (spectrum as a result of scan for entire UV-Visible range).

- Sample cell need to be quartz in UV light measurement, because glass can absorb UV light. But for Visible light measurement (colorimetric) glass cuvettes can be used.

- The sample concentration should be low, and transparent to avoid scattering and beers law deviations.

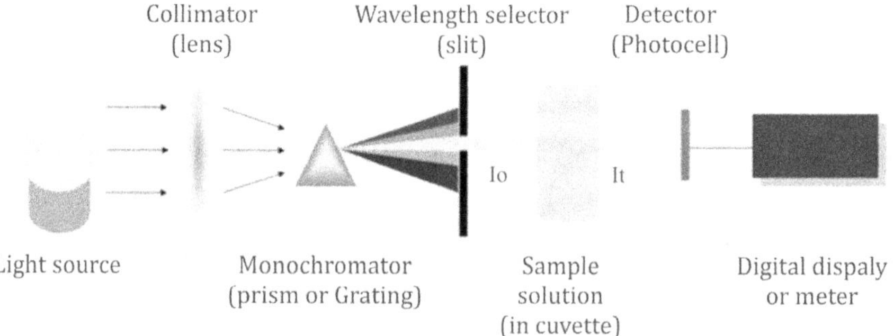

Figure 1.4 Basic Instrumentation of UV-Visible Spectrophotometer.

- Io is the intensity of incident light (monochromatic), I_t is the intensity of transmitted light.

- If Io = I_t sample inactive and indicate no absorption, and molecule structure may not have n and pi electrons.

- If Io is greater than I_t – indicate the reduction of intensity of transmitted light due to absorption of photon energy by the molecular electrons, by the process of electronic excitation.

- Hence Absorbance A = log (Io/I_t) or A = –log T; (where T = It/Io).

The UV Spectrum

For example (2D- UV spectrum) the following UV spectra shows absorption in UV region (190 – 380 nm) indicate the sample is colorless (Figure 1.5).

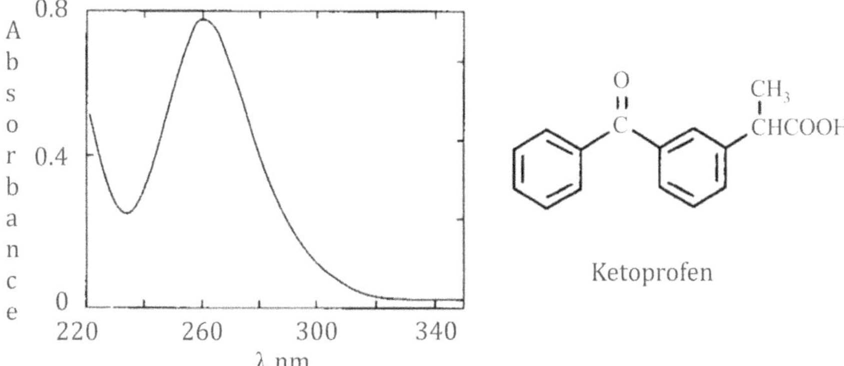

Figure 1.5 UV – Spectrum and UVmax (Lambda max) : Colourless Compound.

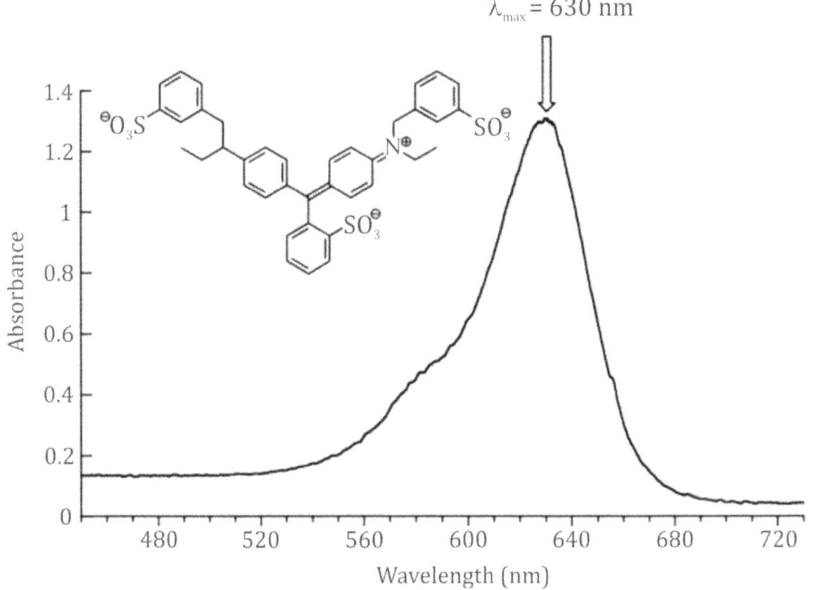

Figure 1.6 UV – Spectrum and absorption maximum: Coloured Compound.

The above UV spectrum is for Colour less sample shows a cut-off wavelength around 340 nm and lambda max of 260 nm. Thus the spectrum shows no absorbance in visible region

- In the same way coloured compound showed absorption maximum at 630 nm, but showed no absorbance in UV region (Figure 1.6).
- Visible spectrum of Coloured sample. Indicate the absorption characteristics of sample in the visible region (400-780 nm).
- The spectrum (Figure 1.7) shows that a spectrum characteristic does not affected by Concentration.

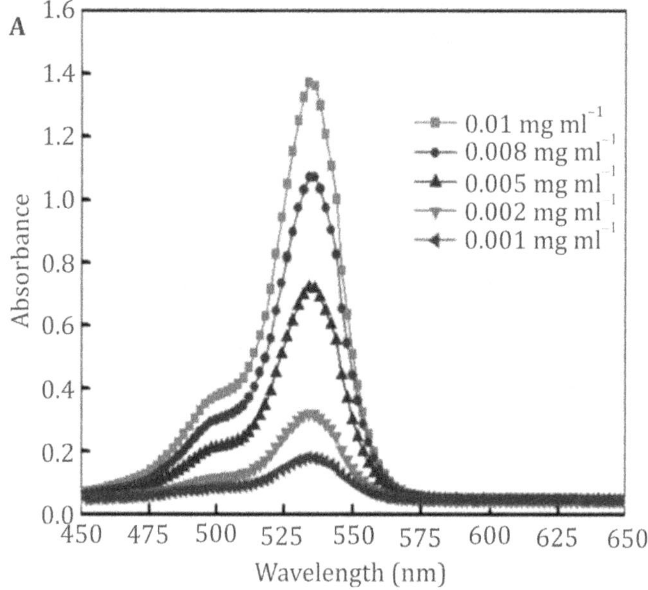

Figure 1.7 UV – Spectrum Vs Concentration (Shows that there is no change in spcetrum chracteristics).

Beer-Lambert Law

- The absorption and Concentration is related by Beer-Lambert law.

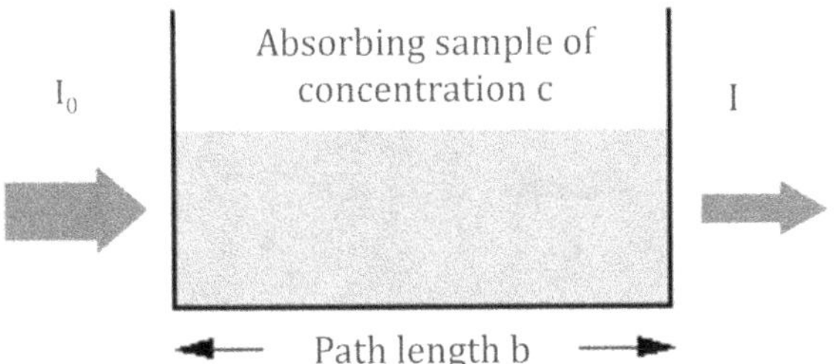

The Beer-Lambert equation shall be expressed as following,

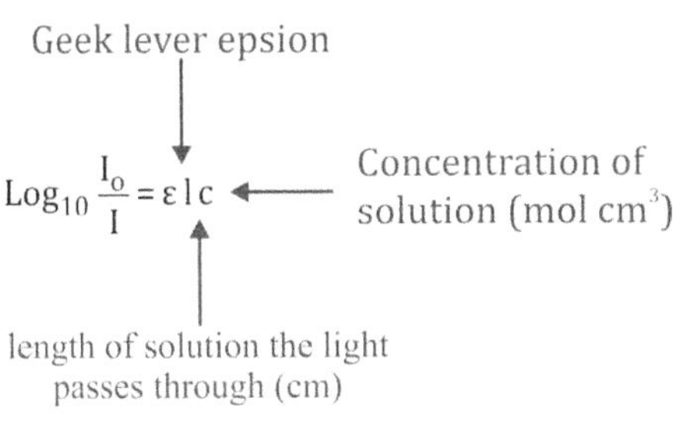

(Or)

$$A = A^{1\%}_{cm}. \; b. \; c$$

Where

- A = Absorbance, (log (Io/I)
- b or l-Path length and c is concentration (g/100 ml),
- A1%cm- the specific absorbance of compound which is constant (it is the absorbance of 1 % w/v solution in 1cm path length).

The above formula is recommended by many pharmacopoeias in quantification of drug in pharmaceutical dosage form, when standard substance is not available.

- The relation between concentration and absorbance is expressed as linearity cure or Beer-Lambert curve. This curve can be used for quantification if both standard and sample available (Figure 1.8).

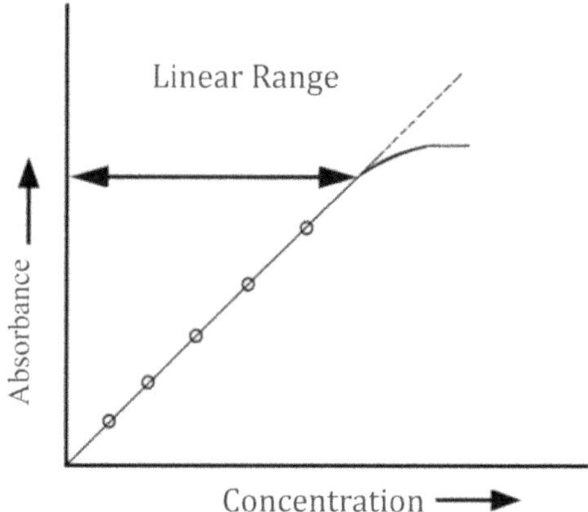

Figure 1.8 Beer-Lambert Plot – Shows the linear relationship between concentration and absorbance to certain limit.

3D UV Spectrum

It is more commonly employed in Chromatography as a function of detection using Photo-diode array detection (PDA). X-axis (wavelength), Y-axis (absorbance), Z axis (time), which can be more conveniently used for kinetic studies. PDA Detection is more commonly employed in stability and degradation of analyte. This detection can give peak purity when coupled with chromatography. This can also predict the response of analyte at different wavelength.

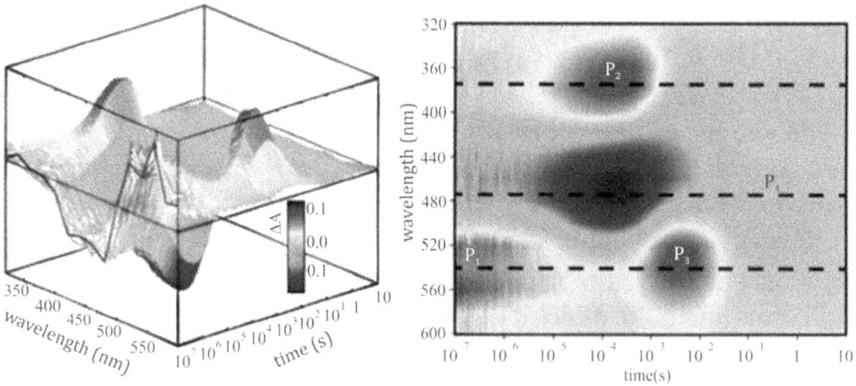

Figure 1.9 3D – UV Visible Spectrum (Example – PDA).

The comparison of absorption spectrum and emission spectrum

- The molecule which possesses more conjugation and exhibit tendency to emit light are called fluorescence. This molecule will have both absorption characteristic spectrum (excitation) and emission characteristic spectrum (emission).

- But emission spectrum will be bathochromic (red shift), it means the spectrum will shift to higher wavelength. The spectrum (Figure 1.9) shows that fluorescence wavelength shifted to higher wavelength than absorption wavelength.

- Maxima of absorption spectrum is excitation wavelength and maxima of emission spectrum is emission wavelength (In fluorimetry)

- If the wavelength shifts to lower wavelength it's called hypsochromic shift. The hyper and hypo chromic shift are used to indicate the absorption to higher and lower value respectively (Figure 1.10). These effects are called auxochrome effect (UV Spectrum nomenclature).

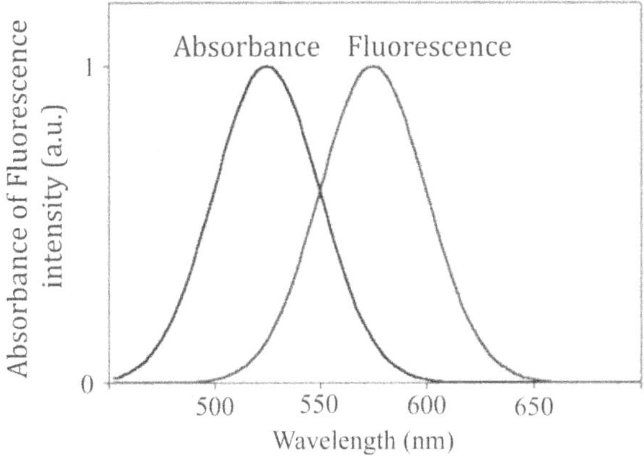

Figure 1.10 Absorption and Emission (Fluorescence) spectrum for an analyte (Stokes shift).

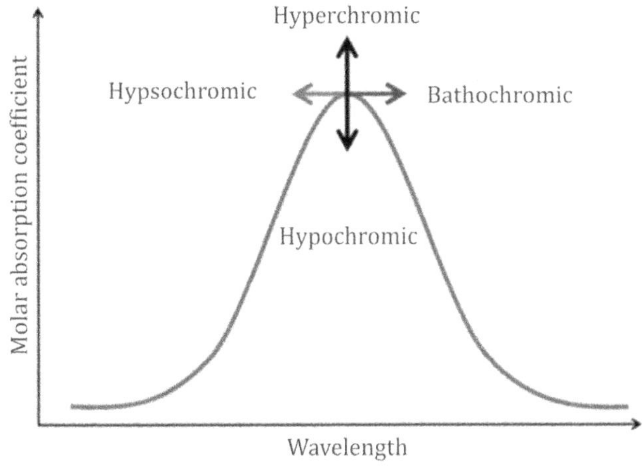

Figure 1.11 Various effect of auxochrome on Absorption maximum (UV-Spectra nomenclature).

All these four effect is seen (Figure 1.10), when there is any change in the following,

- pH,
- solvent,
- scan speed,
- chemical decomposition,
- change in structure,
- isomerism,
- tautomer's

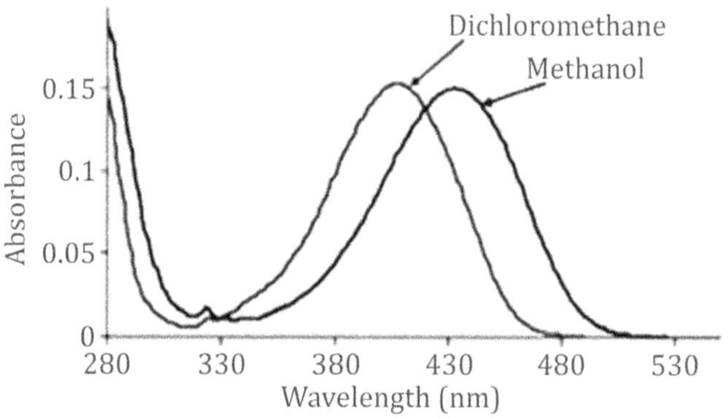

Figure 1.12 Effect of solvent on light absorption of an analyte.

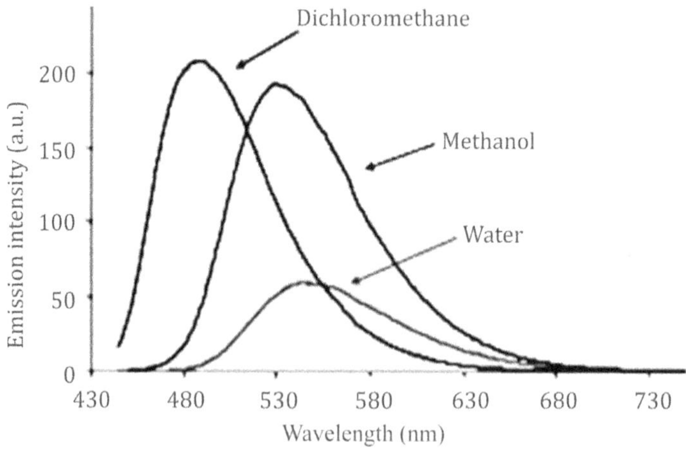

Figure 1.13 Effect of solvent on emission intensity of analyte (Fluorescence).

- The above spectrum (Figure 1.11) shows that there is a bathochromic shift for a molecule when polarity of solvent is increased. (Methanol is polar and dichloromethane is non-polar).

- The relation between polarity of solvent and shift of wavelength depends on the type electronic excitation (nothing but depends on structure and electron involved).

- Usually n- electrons excitation more affected by polar solvent (Hypochromic effect with increase in polarity) and vice versa for pi electrons (Hence, both "positive and negative solvatochromism" is possible)

- In the same way, solvent also affect the emission intensity of an analyte (Figure 1.12).

Solvent Effect and Absorption

Solvato chromism is the ability of a chemical substance to change color due to a change in solvent polarity. Negative solvate chromism corresponds to hypsochromic shift (or blue shift) with increasing solvent polarity. The corresponding bathochromic shift (or red) is termed positive solvatochromism.

In the UV spectrum the absorption from 200 nm to 220 nm,(sliding slope) is due to solvent or , due to both solvent and solute, hence, the wavelength should not be chosen in quantitative analysis. Furthermore, the absorption characteristics also changes in between 200 – 220 nm up on change in solvents. The various solvents and cut-off wavelength are listed in Table 1.2.

So it is always advisable to choose characteristic wavelength beyond the solvent absorption (I.e. above 230 nm). The following overlay spectrum shows the significant difference in the absorbance as well in wavelength for a same compound but in different solvents. It's all due various interactions exist between solute and solvent that ultimately affect the electron transition energies and transition probability. In the below UV-Visible spectrum dotted line (..........) is due to solvent absorption. Solid lines are spectrum of sample with solvent / without solvent effect.

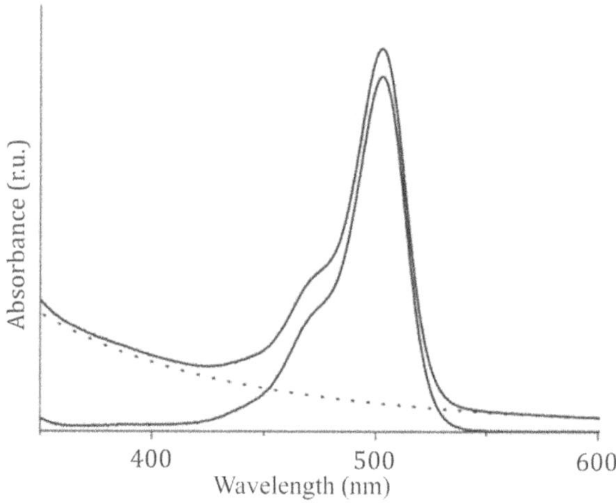

Figure 1.14 Solvent effect on UV-Visible light absorption.

The transparency limit of various UV solvent is given in the below Table 1.2.

Table 1.2 Transparency limit of commonly used Solvent in UV-Visible spectroscopy

Solvent	Cutoff Point (nm)	Solvent	Cutoff Point (nm)[a]
Water	200	Dichloromethane	233
Ethanol (95%)	205	Butyl ether	235
Acetonitrile	210	Chloroform	245
Cyclohexane	210	Ethyl proprionate	255
Cyclopentane	210	Methyl formate	260
Heptane	210	Carbon tetrachloride	265
Hexane	210	N,N-Dimethylformamide	270
Methanol	210	Benzene	280
Pentane	210	Toluene	285
Isopropyl alcohol	210	m-Xylene	290
Isooctane	215	Pyridine	305
Dioxane	220	Acetone	330
Diethyl ether	220	Bromoform	360
Glycerol	220	Carbon disulfide	380
1,2-Dichloroethane	230	Nitromethane	380

[a]Wavelength at which the absorbance is unity for a 1-cm cell, with water as the reference.

Structure and Spectrum Characteristics

- The absorption spectrum shape and pattern is depends on the structure, so that UV spectrum is considered as one of the identification tools in modern analytical chemistry.

- The electrons and bonds and their position (electronic configuration) determine the spectrum characteristics.

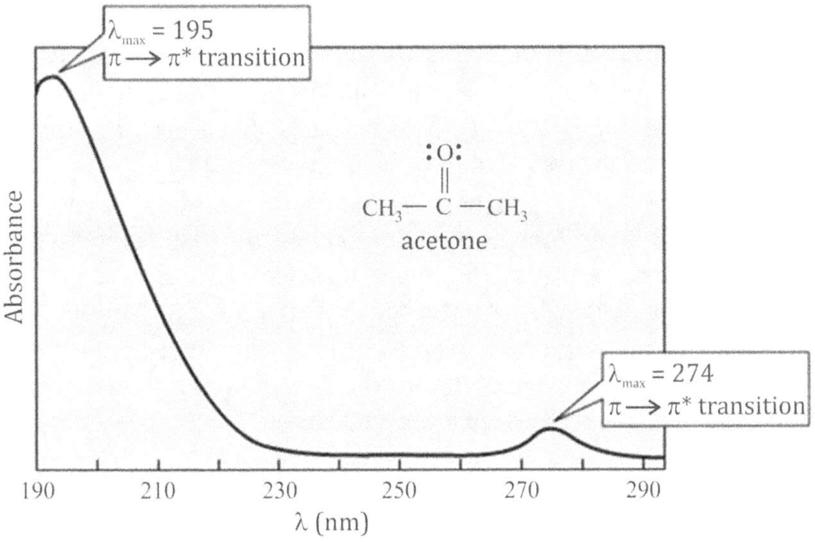

Figure 1.15 UV-Spectrum of Acetone.

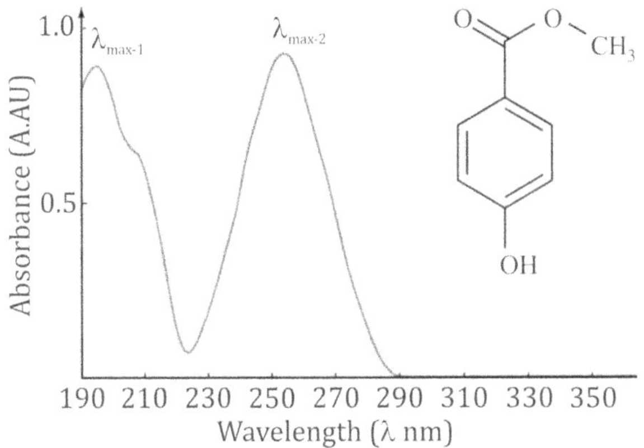

Figure 1.16 UV-Spectrum of aromatic ester.

1. For example above two spectrum are not similar indicate the compounds are different

2. Acetone UV spectrum (Figure 1.12) two maxima, one at 195 nm (for pi electron transition) and one at 274 nm (n' electron transitions), but the intensity for pi' (195 nm) is more than n' electron (274 nm). It indicate that the transition probability for pi is more in the structure when compare to n' electron. As a

result, the molar absorptivity (Epsilon value) will be more for Pi′ and less for n′ electron).

3. When look into the second spectrum (Figure 1.13), the intensity of peak absorption is increased due to conjugation. Furthermore, lambda max increases due to conjugation.

4. Hence the conjugation in structure will have greater effect on transition energy as well in wavelength absorbed.

5. The following UV spectrum is one more example for different transition in a molecule and its effect on UV spectrum. Where Pi to Pi is stronger and n′ to pi is weaker. So always pi to pi transition yield greater absorbance than n′ to pi transitions.

6. Pi to pi transitions always occur in low wavelength when compare to n′ electrons due to the fact the energy of electron is in the order of Sigma > pi > n′ electrons.

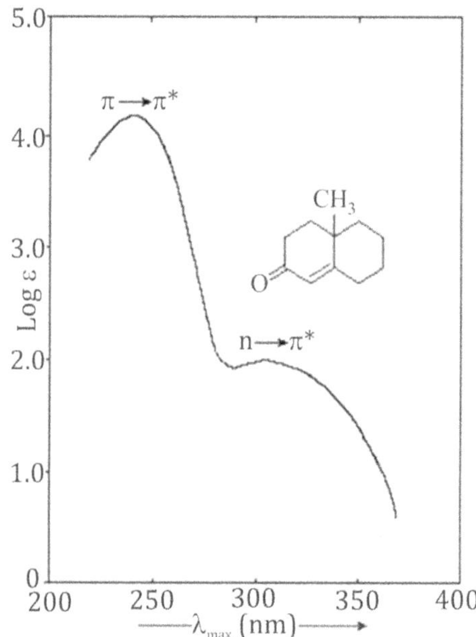

Figure 1.17 UV-Spectrum of Naphthalenone hexahydro methyl.

1. The following overlay UV- Visible spectrum shows the effect of conjugation on UV-spectrum and number maxima in spectrum characteristics. As the conjugation increase in the structure the spectrum moves towards higher wavelength (bathochromic effect).

2. Number of maxima is also increases as number conjugation increases.

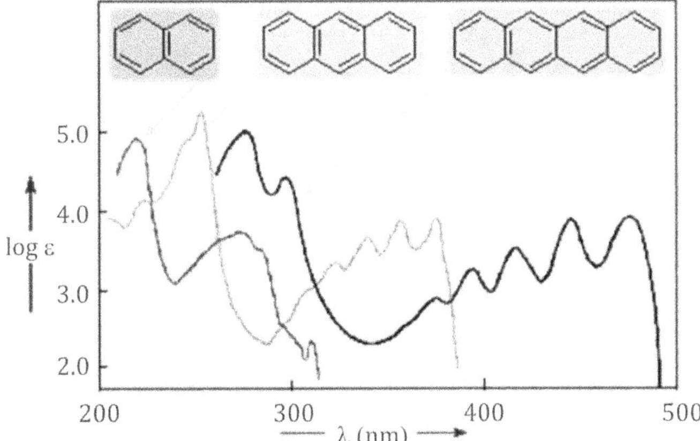

Figure 1.18 Effect of Conjugation on UV-Visible spectrum Characteristics.

1. **Cross Conjugation:** The below two structures are similar but differ in the electronic transition pattern as well in UV spectrum due to the n' electron contribute addition transition. Below structure also an example for cross conjugation.

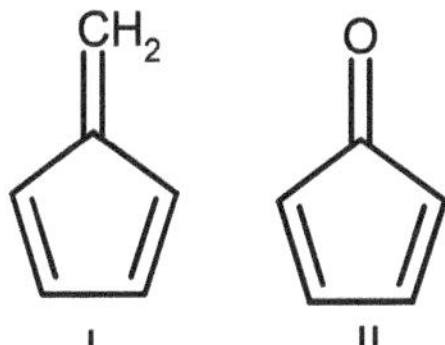

Auxochrome effect: The below spectrum of quinones, shows the comparison of similar structures with same chromophoric system (conjugated system responsible for light absorption), but differ in substitution at NH2 group. Thus the substitution on chromophoric system has effect on both lambda max and absorbance (Figure 1.14 and Figure 1.15)

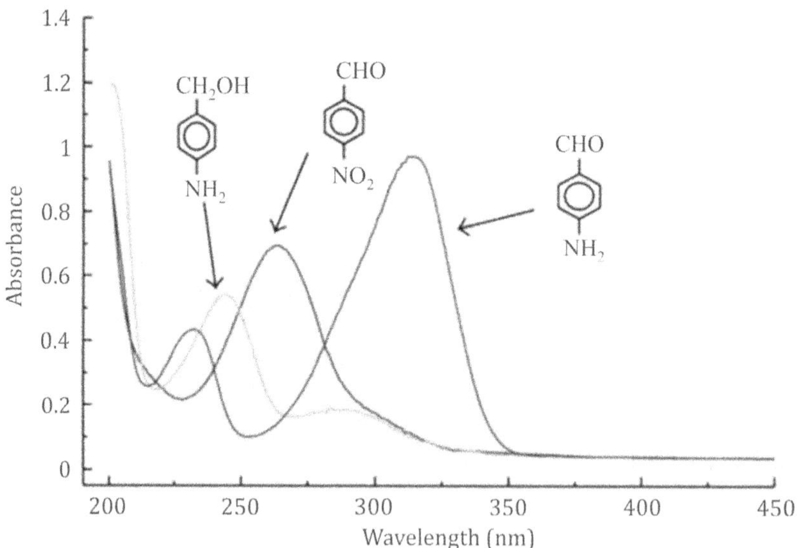

Figure 1.19 Auxochrome effect of UV-Visible spectrum Characteristics (Solvent: DMSO).

Figure 1.20 Auxochrome effect of UV-Visible spectrum Characteristics.

Order of Conjugation: The imidazole carboxylic acid (Figure 1.16) represents the order of conjugation in UV spectrum characteristics. The UV spectrum move higher wavelength when there is more conjugation. You can observe the change in the double bond position in imidazole nucleus of the structure.

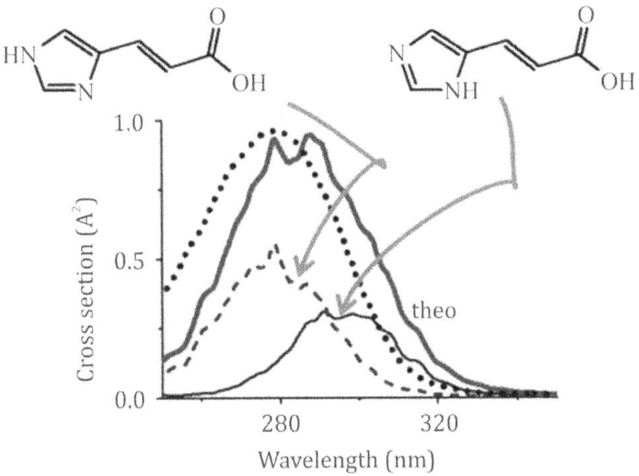

Figure 1.21 Effect of Order of Conjugation in UV-Visible spectrum Characteristics.

Position of Auxochrome in Chromophore: The below structure represent the importance of Auxochrome in benzene and their UV light absorption pattern. The presence of amine group may have significant effect on Lambda max and light absorption intensity. The ortho position in the below structure may contribute intra molecular hydrogen bonding and produce a addition cyclic residue to the structure as well as it also produce, inductive effect.

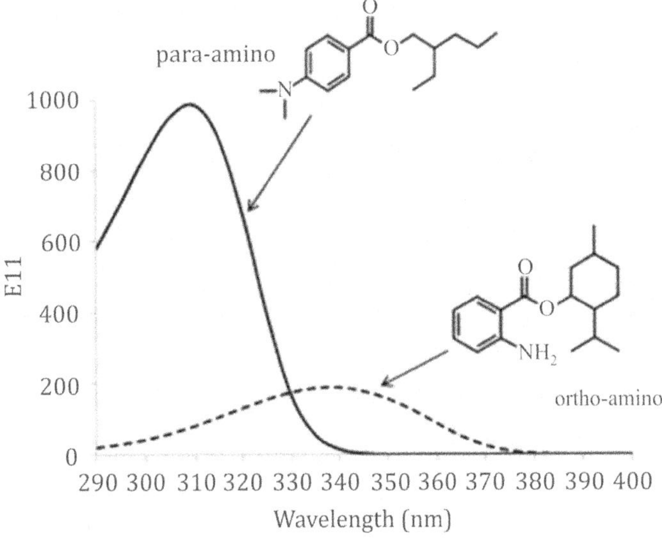

Figure 1.22 Effect of Auxochrome position on UV-Visible spectrum Characteristics.

Cis - Trans Isomerism and UV spectrum: The azobenzene is the best example of conformation transformation due to UV light and both are inter-convertible.

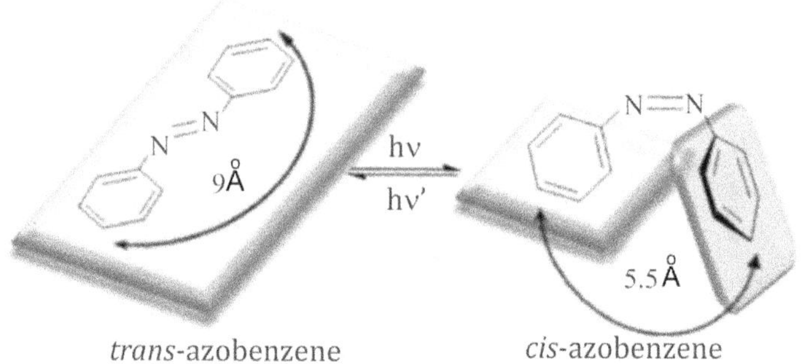

trans-azobenzene   cis-azobenzene

Like a C=C double bond, the azobenzenes have two geometric isomers (Z/E) around the N=N double bond, the *trans* isomer (E) is ~12 kcal·mol⁻¹ more stable than the *cis* isomer (Z). The energy barrier of the photoexcited state is ~23 kcal·mol⁻¹, such that the *trans* isomer is predominant in the dark at room temperature. This energy barrier make different UV spectrum for trans (high intense) and Cis isomer.

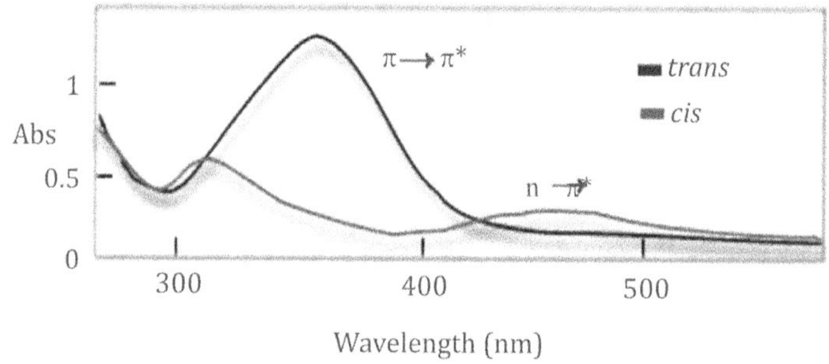

Figure 1.23 Effect of *Cis /Trans* isomer on UV-Visible spectrum Characteristics.

Keto-enol tautomer's in UV spectrum: The following figure shows the UV spectrum for same structure but exist in different tautomerism. B is Keto' form. A and C are enol form. For enol' structure spectrum is moved to higher wavelength due to induction of conjugation and extension of conjugation. Where as in structure B' both benzene is isolated not in conjugation.

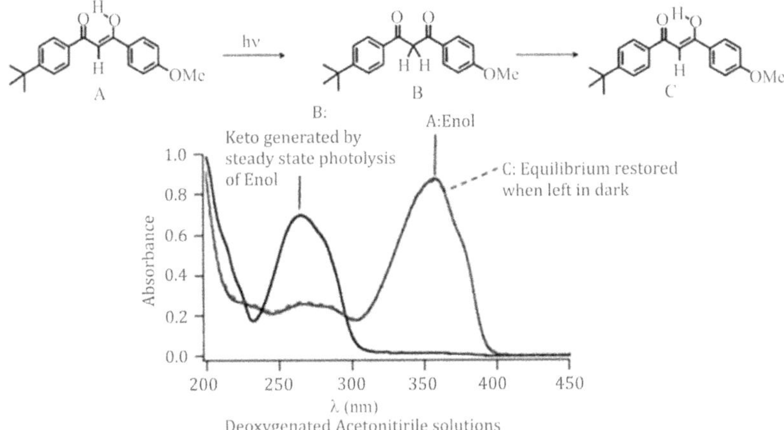

Figure 1.24 Effect of tautomerism on UV-Visible spectrum Characteristics.

Identification of Compound by UV Spectrum

For example: Ibuprofen, the following figure 1.19, shows the three UV spectra overlapped indicated that three (a, b, c) are same, as they have same UV spectrum and fingerprint matching of absorption characteristics.

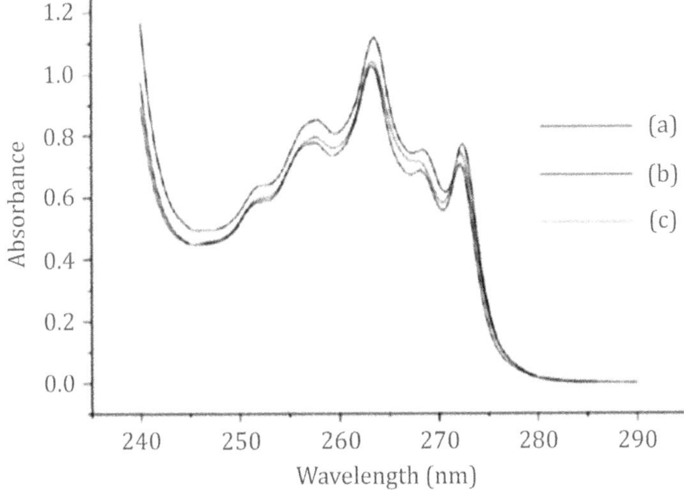

Figure 1.25 Overlay UV- Spectra of three different batch Ibuprofen samples.

The following UV spectrum (Figure 1.20) of four chrysene derivatives indicates that substitution (Auxochrome) will have impact on UV spectrum fingerprint (pattern of absorption), so no two derivatives of same chemical class would have same spectrum

Identification of degradation by UV spectrum

The degradation by UV spectrum can be identified by three ways

1. **Change in absorption pattern and fingerprint (shift of maxima, appearance and disappearance of maxima, change in cut off wavelength):** The following UV spectrum (Figure 1.21) shows the change in absorption pattern of compound after 90 minutes.

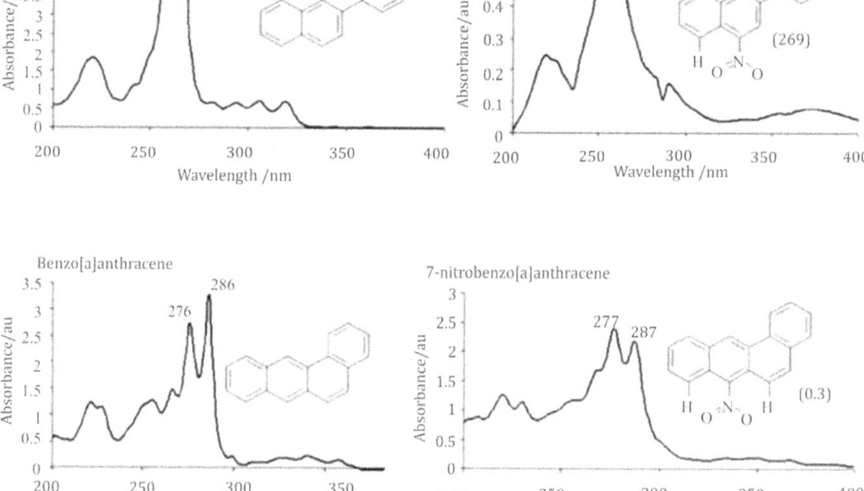

Figure 1.26 Overlay UV- Spectra of four derivatives of chrysene.

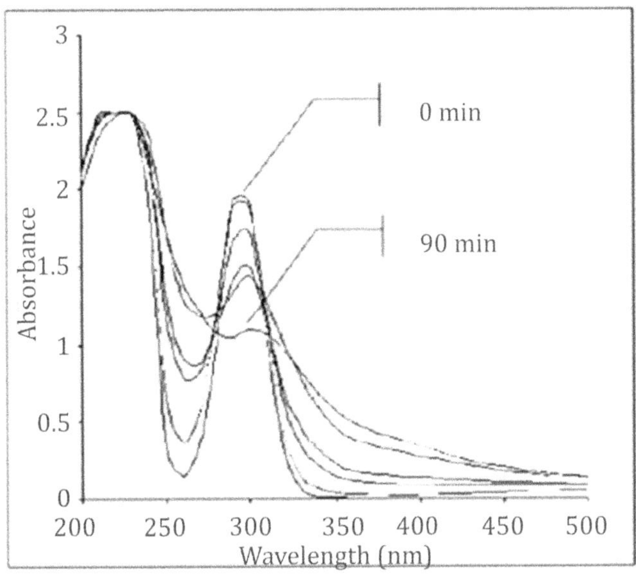

Figure 1.27 Overlay UV- Spectra of decomposed product at different time intervals.

2. **Change in absorption (at maxima and valley):** The UV spectrum (Figure 1.21) shows that there is an absolute shift of UVmax and valley point with respect to time.

3. **Change in shape of the spectrum and AUC of the UV spectrum:** The UV spectrum (Figure 1.22) shows the change in AUC and shape of UV spectrum up on degradation.

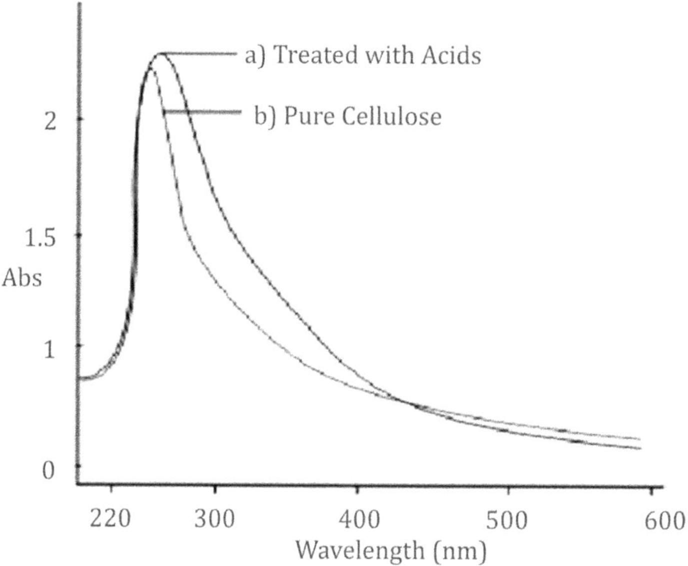

Figure 1.28 Overlay UV- Spectra of decomposed cellulose (Acid treated) and Pure Cellulose.

Differentiation of benzenoid and quinonoid by UV spectrum: It is more common with indication, at different pH the indicator colour will be different so the UV-visible spectrum also different for same indicator at different pH. The following is the example (Figure 1.22) of Phenol red indicator; we can observe the shift of spectrum between acid form and base form.

Isosbestic point: However, there is a different absorption pattern for acidic /basic or ionized or unionized form of a chemical species, there a wavelength in which two compounds or different forms will have same absorbance. This particular wavelength is called as isosbestic point (Figure 1.22). The isosbestic point and its relevant absorbance are very import in simultaneous or multicomponent analysis (Q-analysis or absorbance ratio method).

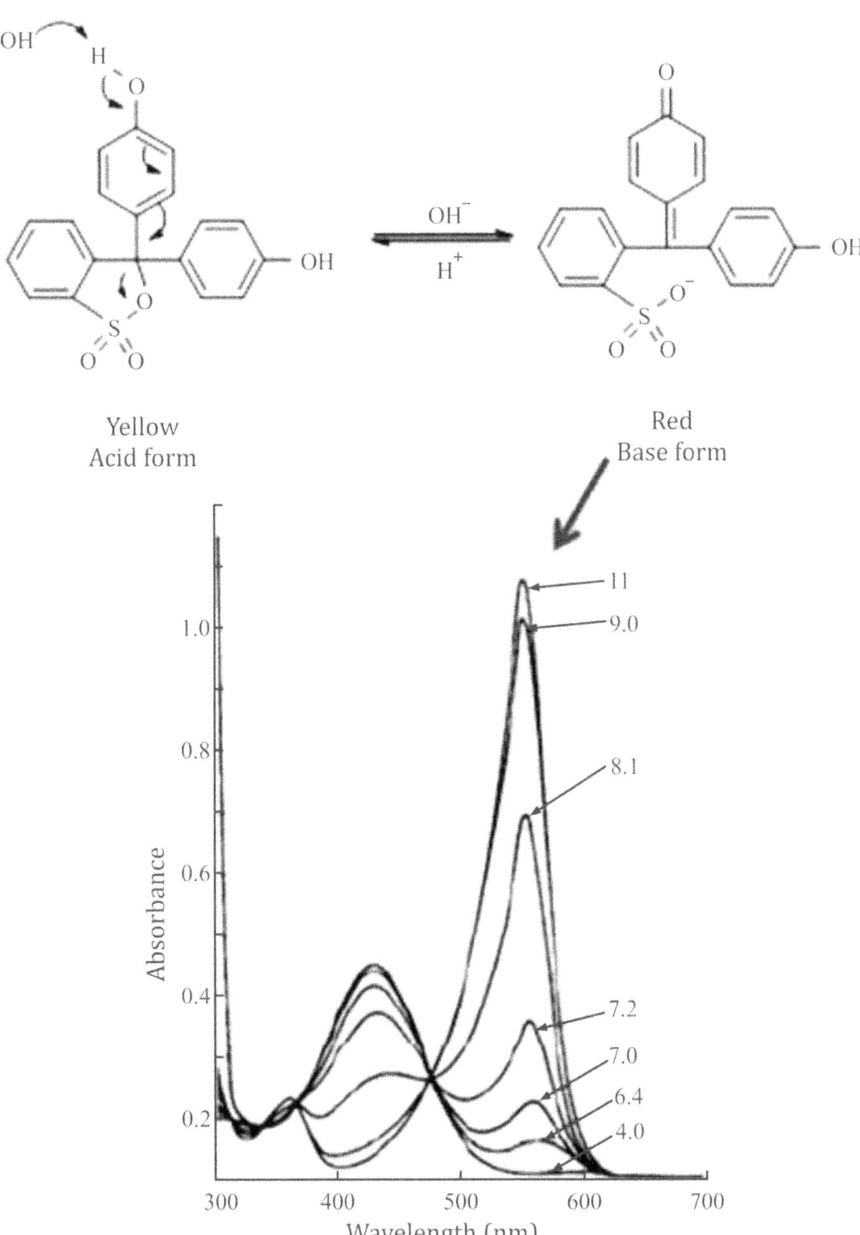

Figure 1.29 Overlay UV - Spectra of Phenol red indicators (at different pH).

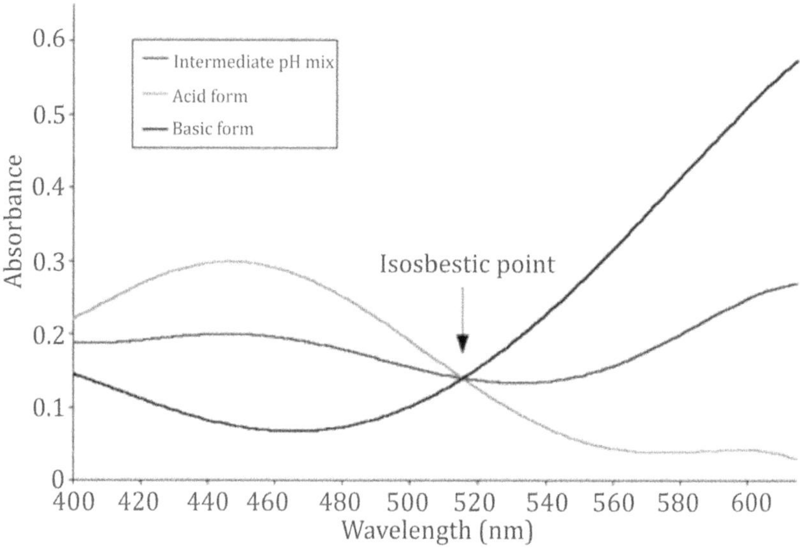

Figure 1.30 Overlay UV - Spectra of a compound at different pH (Isosbestic point).

Differentiation of ionized and unionized form of compounds (ex. Barbiturates): The following UV spectrum (Figure 1.23) represents the example of ionized and unionized spectrum of Barbiturate. It can be noticed that maxima was absent unionized form of barbiturate (A), Where Spectrum B' and C' are other ionized form of barbiturate. So, pH of solvent in quantitative analysis is very important factor for certain drugs.

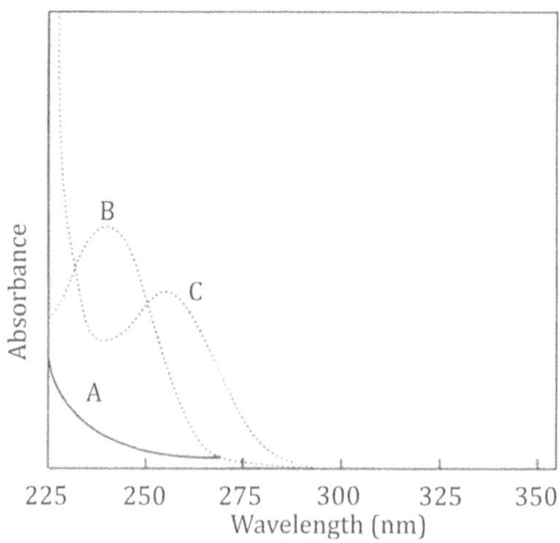

Figure 1.31 Overlay UV- Spectra of Barbiturate (A: unionized; B &C are ionized at different proportions).

Determination of pKa by UV-spectrum

When there is a pH dependent absorbance changes takes place for a molecule, it is possible to determine the pKa by UV spectroscopy. The following figure 1.32 shows, the change absorbance with respect to change in pH values for isolapachol. The pKa was found to be 5.75 for isopachol

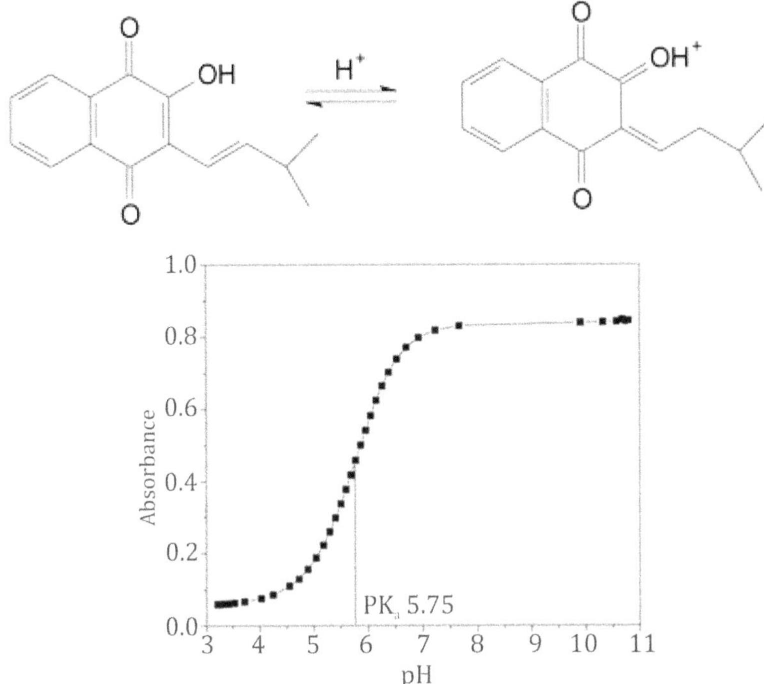

Figure 1.32 Effect of pH on UV- Visible light absorbance.

pKa is the pH in which both ionized and unionized forms are equal. That exhibit direct relation in absorbance value.

Use of UV spectrum in Immune mediated complex: The following spectrum (Figure 1.33) shows the assay relies upon gold nanoparticles (AuNPs) based complex in the immunoreactions of antigen and antibody that can induce the aggregation of antibody-functionalized AuNPs. The UV spectrum shows significant shift in absorbance as well in wavelength to indicate the presence or absence of complex.

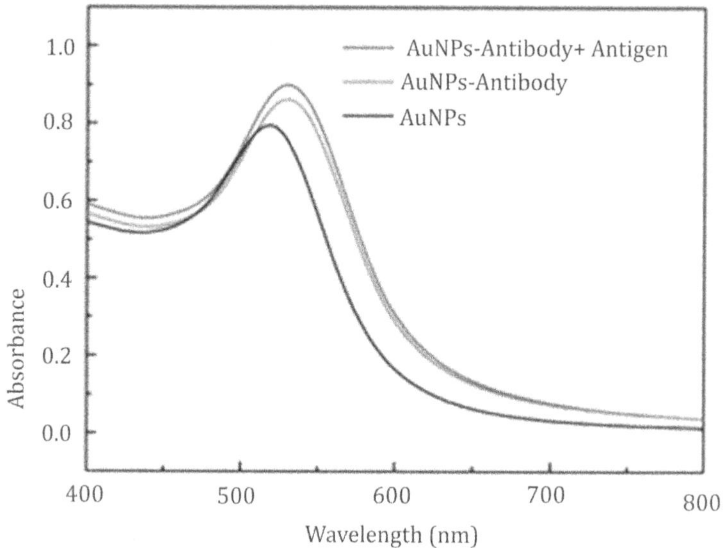

Figure 1.33 Overlay UV spectra in Immune mediated recation and its complex.

Identification of natural pigments: The UV spectrum is the good indicator to identify the natural pigments. The following figure 1.34 shows the UV- visible spectrum of several natural compounds which are distinct in their absorption characteristics.

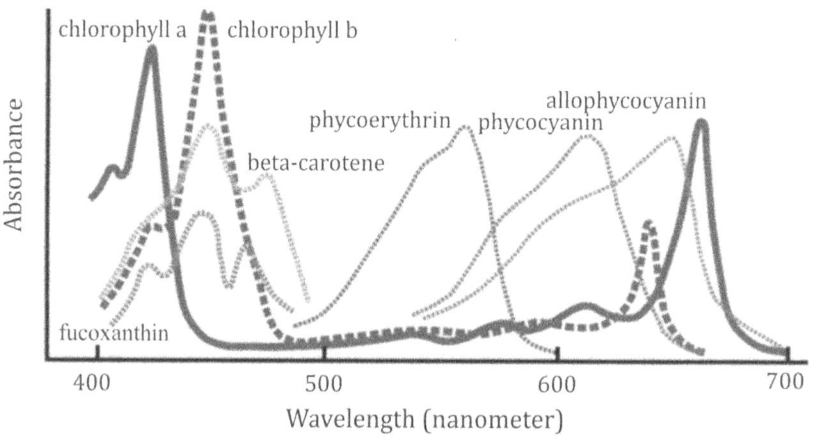

Figure 1.34 Overly UV spectra of natural pigments.

Detection of impurity by UV spectrum: There is a chance for predicting the presence of impurity (preferably at moderate level of concentration). The following UV spectrum (Figure 1.35) shows considerable shift of 2 nm for both maxima (275 nm) and Valley (248 nm) along with the maxima effect below 246 nm. This may be because of the presence of potential dissolved impurities.

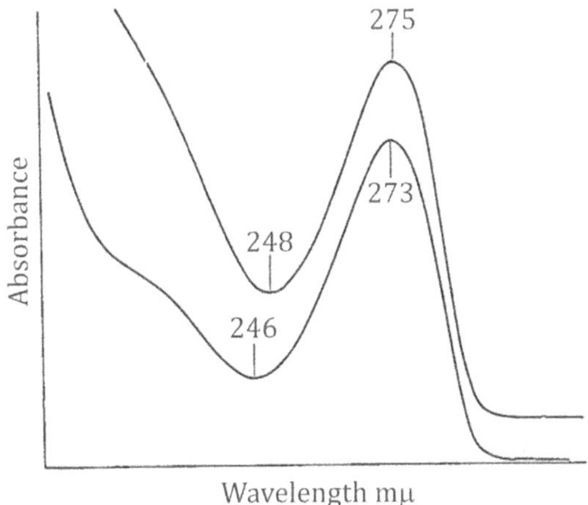

Figure 1.35 Detection of impurity by UV spectra.

Identification of Active pharmaceutical ingredients in Dosage form: It is done by comparison of Sample UV spectrum with reference UV spectrum (finger print matching; Figure 1.36). The excipient effects in UV absorption below 250 nm have to be considered or placebo correction may be required. The spectra A and C are sample, B is standard.

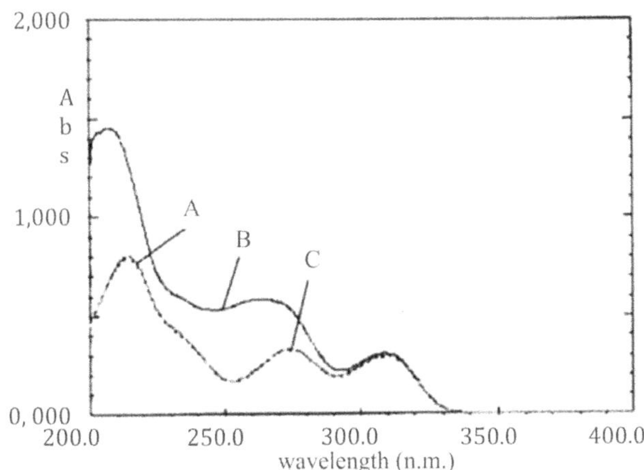

Figure 1.36 Identification of API in dosage form by UV spectrum.

Identification mixture using standards: If a UV spectrum is considered as mixture of two drugs (A and B), then the overlay spectra of pure drugs A and B and the mixture C can give us the information regarding authentication of drugs in the mixture. In the below figure 1.37, A and B are UV spectrum of pure drugs, where C (dotted line) is the mixture. The spectrum of C can be matched with spectrum of both A and B.

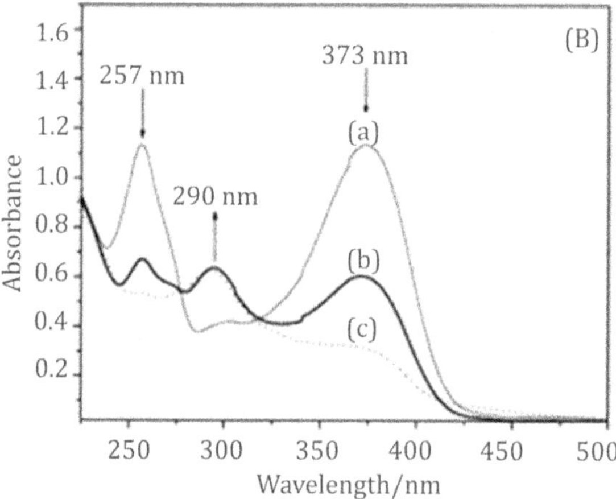

Figure 1.37 Identification of mixture using standard by UV spectra overlay.

WOODWARD RULES (Rules in calculation of UV max (λ max) for chemical compounds)

"As lambda (λ) max increases that indicate the compound structure has more conjugation, with increase in pi-electron density. This lambda (λ) max vary from structure to structure (Figure 1.38 and 1.39) even with same number of double bond and conjugation, Lambda max (λ) is depends on position of the double bond rather than degree and number of double bond"

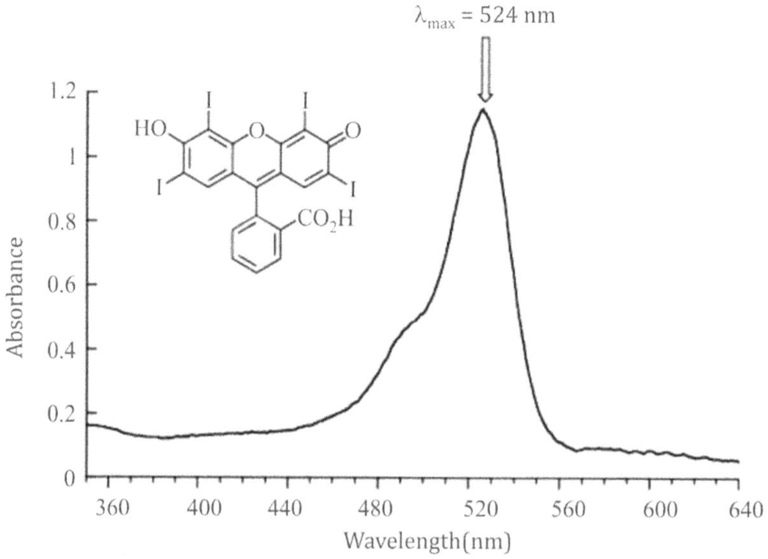

Figure 1.38 Determination of lambda (λ) max in UV Spectrum.

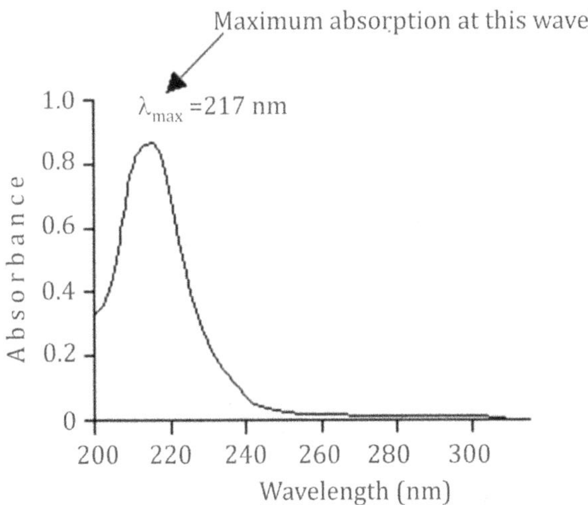

Figure 1.39 Maximum Absorption (λ max) in UV absorption of diene compounds.

'**WOODWARD- FIESER RULES**: Each type of diene or triene system is having a certain fixed value at which absorption takes place; this constitutes the *Base value or Parent value*. The contribution made by various alkyl substituents or ring residue, double bond extending conjugation and polar groups such as –Cl, -Br etc are added to the basic value to obtain λ_{max} for a particular compound'.

Descriptors used in (λ max) calculations of 1, 3 butadiene chromophore

$$H_2C=CH-CH=CH_2$$

Core chromophore

NOTE: *Only conjugated dienes are considered to account for woodward rules for prediction (λ max).1, 3 –butadiene system is essentioal to consider the structure for woodward rule.*

Table 1.3 Basic understanding in Woodward rule for calculation of λ max

Descriptors	Definition	Structure	Value
Homoannular Diene	Cyclic diene having conjugated double bonds in same ring		253 nm

Table 1.3 *contd...*

Descriptors	Definition	Structure	Value
Hetero annular Diene	Cyclic diene having conjugated double bonds in different rings (A and B)	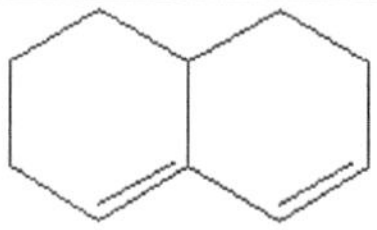	215 nm
Endocyclic double bond	Double bond present in a ring	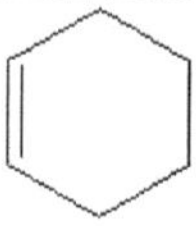	Not considered. It's a part of basic value
Exocyclic double bond	Double bond in which one of the doubly bonded atoms is a part of a ring system.	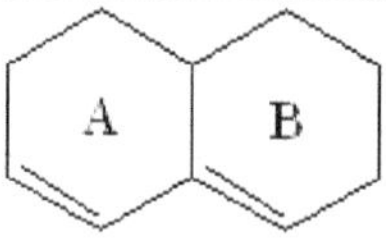 A B Here Ring A has one exocyclic and endocyclic double bond. Ring B has only one endocyclicdouble bond	5 nm
Addition Conjugation	Addition one double to the basic Chromophore (diene)	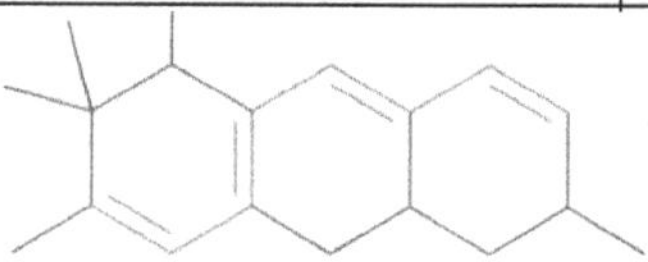 This molecule has two addition conjugation apart from diene (basic)	Each additional conjugation = 30 nm
Cross conjugation	Addition conjugation which is branched	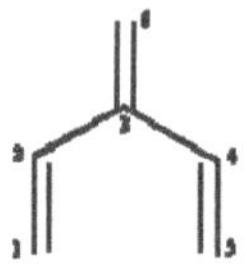 I 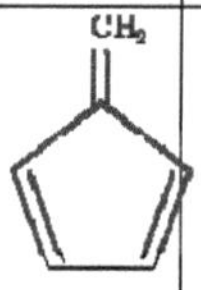 II The above structure the additional conjugation not considered as addition conjugation.	0 nm

(A) Calculation of λ max for the given 1, 3 butadiene structures using Woodward Fieser Rule

Table 1.4 Calculation of λ max for the given 1, 3 butadiene structures using Woodward Fieser Rule

Descriptors	Value to be considered in calculation (in nm) – Substituent effect (Auxochrome)
Homoannular (cisoid)	253 nm
Heteroannular (transoid)	215 nm
Acyclic diene	217 nm
Double bond extending conjugation	30 nm
Alkyl substituent or ring residue	5 nm
Exocyclic double bond	5 nm
-OC(O)CH$_3$	0 nm
-OR	6 nm
-Cl, -Br	5 nm
-NR$_2$	60 nm
-SR	30 nm
Phenyl ring	75 nm

λ max = BAERS (B+A+E+R+S)

- *B*- Basic value (such as Hetero annular or Homoannular or acyclic)
- *A* – additional conjugation
- *E* – exocyclic double bond
- *R* – Ring residues
- *S* – substitution on the conjugated chain (not on other part of structure)

Additional Conjugation

Bonds in alternative position are considered to be extending conjugation. In the below structure the bond between C6 and C7 is isolated from diene, so it cannot be considered as extending conjugation or addition conjugation. **Thus it has 0 (zero) value in calculation.**

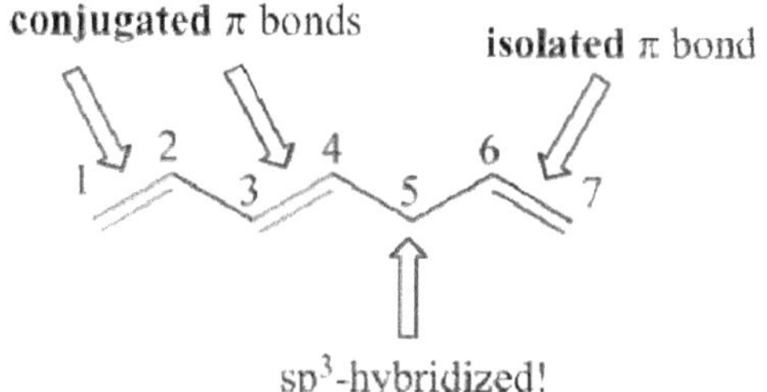

In the below structure, there is a ONE extended or additional conjugation to diene. So (1 × 30 nm) 30 nm has to be added in the calculation.

H_2C ⟍⟍ ⟋⟋ ⟍⟍ CH_2

Exocyclic Double Bond

- The above structure has both heteroannulardiene and homoannulardiene. But basic value has be based on homoannulardiene.

- The exocyclic double bond has to be calculated based on the position, thus above structure has THREE exocyclic double bond (3 × 5 = 15 nm)

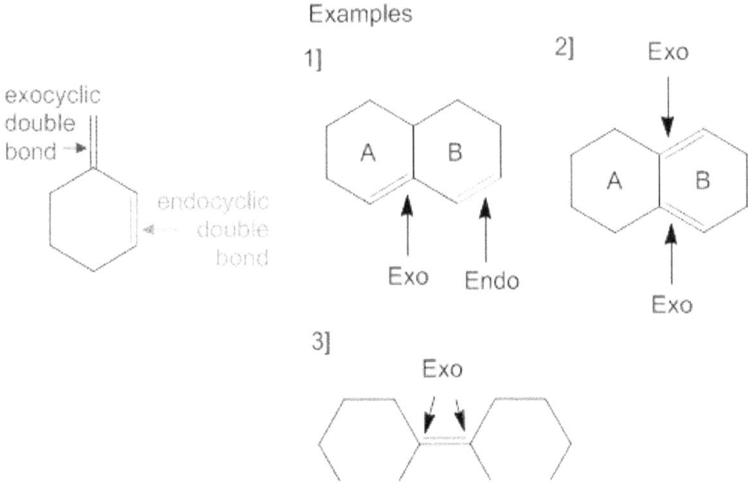

The above figure differentiates between exocyclic (shown in red) and endocyclic (shown in green) double bonds.

1. In example 1, the double bond present within ring A is exocyclic to ring B as it is attached to an atom which is shared between ring A and ring B, while the double bond present in ring B is not connected to any ring A atoms and is within just one ring, hence making it endocyclic.

2. In example 2, both double bonds are present within ring B with connections to shared carbon atoms with ring A, making both the double bonds exocyclic.

3. In example 3, there is a single double bond which is exocyclic at two points to two different rings. In such a case, the influence would be 2 times + 5 nm (i.e + 10 nm).

"Solvent effects: *Since the conjugated diene base is relatively non-polar, contribution due to different solvents is very minor and can be ignored in most cases".*

Ring Residue

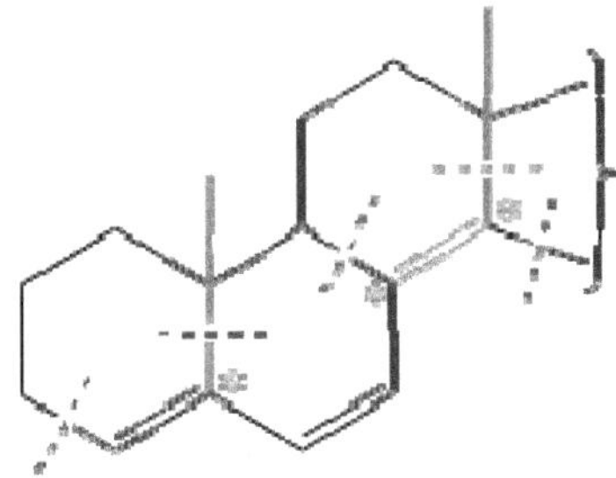

It is the number of bond cleavage to be done on the ring structure to isolate the entire conjugated chain, thus above structure has five ring residue (5 × 5 = 25 nm) and 25 nm has to added in the calculation

Substitution on the Structure

In the below structure all substitution (R) are attached with the carbon which involved in the conjugation, hence value has to added (Auxochrome effect) in the calculation.

In the below steroidal compounds, substitutions ar C2 and C4 are not considered, as they are not a part of conjugated system, thus the below structure has no substitution value in calculation. But has ring residue, exocyclic and basic values.

Example of Calculation

Absorption maximum : 214 + 20 + 5 = 239 nm

Heteroannular diene : 214
alkyl substituents 4 × 5 = 20
exocyclic double bond : 5

Homoannular diene : 253
alkyl substituents : 4 × 5
exocyclic double bond : 2 × 5
Absorption maximum : 253 + 20 + 10 = 283 nm

Example 1:

Basic value (acyclic)	Acyclic diene	217
Additional extended conjugation	--	0
Exocyclic double bond	--	0
Ring residue	Not a cyclic compound	0
Substitution	3 alkyl (3 × 5)	15
TOTAL		**232 nm**

Example 2:

	Homoannular	253
Basic value (acyclic)		
Additional extended conjugation	--	0
Exocyclic double bond	--	0
Ring residue	2 residues (2×5)	10 nm
Substitution	--	0
TOTAL		**263 nm**

Example 3:

Table 1.5 λ max for structural futures

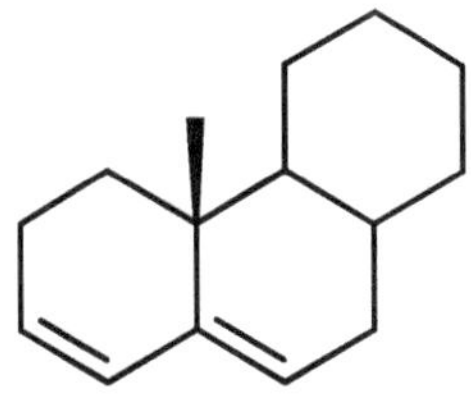

Basic value (acyclic)	Heteroannular	215
Additional extended conjugation	--	0
Exocyclic double bond	One (1 × 5)	5
Ring residue	3 residues (3 × 5)	15 nm
Substitution	--	0
TOTAL		**235 nm**

Example 4:

Basic value (acyclic)	Homoannular	253
Additional extended conjugation	--	0
Exocyclic double bond	One (1 × 5)	5
Ring residue	3 residues (3 × 5)	15 nm
Substitution	1 (isopropyl) alkyl group	5 nm
TOTAL		**278 nm**

Other examples:

Diene Example #1:

Calc. λ_{max} = 214 (acyclic base) + 5 (alkyl auxochrome at C_3) + 5 (alkyl auxochrome at C_4) = 224 nm

One way to identify an auxochrome is to draw a loop around the entire conjugated system (including extending olefins) and then add hash marks across all bonds attached to the loop. The hash marks define auxochrome attachments.

Diene Example #2:

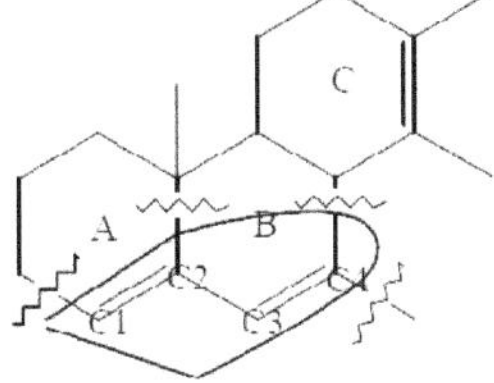

Calc. λ_{max} =   214 (heteroannular since two pi bonds are not in the same ring) + 20 (5 + 5 + 5 + 5 = 20, for each of the alkyl or ring auxochromes attached to C_1, C_2, C_4, and C_4) + 5 (pi bond of C_1-C_2 is exocyclic to ring B) = 239 nm

Diene Example #3:

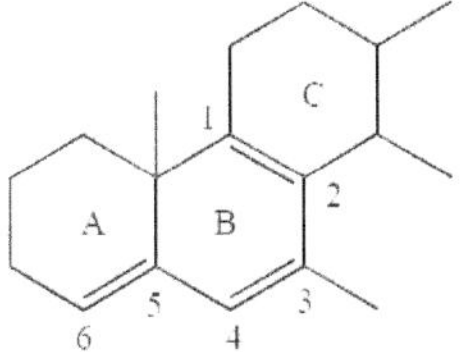

Calc. λ_{max} =   253 (choose diene with highest base value. pi bonds C_{1-2} and C_{3-4} are within same ring. so homoannular base should be selected) + 30 (C_{5-6} pi bond is conjugated to diene and is therefore an extending diene) + 5 (C_{5-6} is exocyclic to ring B) + 30 (5 + 5 + 5 + 5 + 5 + 5 = 30, for the alkyl or ring auxochromes at C_1. C_1, C_2, C_3, C_5, and C_6) = 318 nm

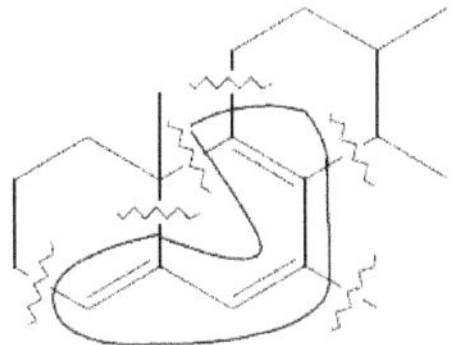

(b)   Calculation of λ max for unsaturated carbonyl compounds

The unsaturated carbonyl compounds (C=O) still considered as conjugated system, so the same method of calculation can be used, with little modification in basic value and residue and substitution values.

Cyclic Unsaturated Carbonyl System

Cyclopentenone   Cyclohexenone

Base value:

(a) Acyclic α, β unsaturated ketones   =   214 nm

(b) 6 membered cyclic α, β unsaturated ketones   =   215 nm

(c) 5 membered cyclic α, β unsaturated ketones   =   202 nm

(d) α, β unsaturated aldehydes   =   210 nm

(e) α, β unsaturated carboxylic acids & esters   =   195 nm

Acyclic unsaturated carbonyl system

Extended Conjugation

R = H = Aldehyde = 240 nm
R = Alkyl = Ketone = 245 nm
R = OAlkyl = Ester = 225 nm

Auxochrome value to be added to basic value of unsaturated carbonyl system in calculation of λ max.

Auxochrome	Alpha	Beta	Gamma	delta
OH or	35	30	--	50
OR (-OCH3)	35	30	17	31
Br	25	30	--	--
Cl	15	12	--	--

CH3 or Any alkyl group	10	12	18	18
Ring residue	10	12	18	18
-OCOR	6	6	6	6
NR2	--	95	--	--

NOTE: Alpha, beta, delta position is assigned only to conjugated carbon system.

Formula

λ max = BAERS (B+A+E+R+S)

- B - Basic value (such as acyclic or cyclopentanone or hexanone)
- A – additional conjugation
- E – exocyclic double bond
- R – Ring residues(different value based on the position like alpha, beta etc)
- S – substitution on the conjugated chain (not on other part of structure)

Basic value (acyclic)	**Cyclohexanone**	**215**
Additional extended conjugation	01	30
Exocyclic double bond	One (1 × 5)	5
Ring residue	12 (beta) + 18 (delta)	30 nm
Substitution	--	0 nm
TOTAL		**280 nm**

Other illustrated Examples

Enone Example #1:

Calc. λ_{max} =   215 (cyclohexenone base) + 30
(extending conjugation) + 5
(α,β olefin is exocyclic to ring
B) + 12 (β auxochrome) − 36
(2 δ auxochromes) = 298 nm

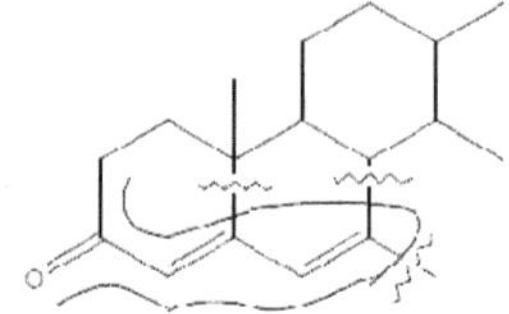

Benzoyl Example #1:

Calc. λ_{max} =   246 (Benzoyl Base,
where Z is the aliphatic methyl group) +
3 (o auxochrome) + 3 (m auxochrome)
= 252 nm

Benzoyl Example # 2:

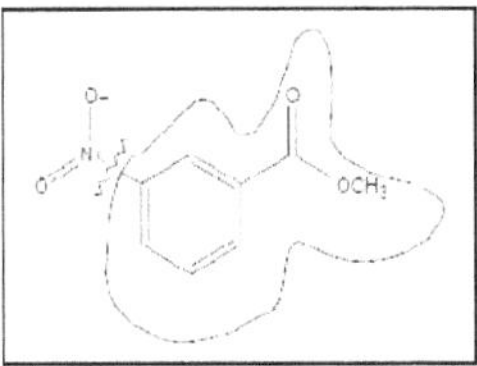

Calc. λ_{max} =   230 (Benzoyl Base, where Z is O-R in this ester functionality) + ?
(There is no value listed for a *meta* nitro group.)

> **230 nm**. The rules are not perfect. They do not allow you to make predictions for all compounds, not even all the simple ones. The best you can predict in this situation is that the observed λ_{max} should be greater than 230 nm. After all, the nitro group contains a π bond that extends the length of the conjugated π system. And if nothing else, you know that greater conjugation means longer wavelength λ_{max}.

(C) λ max Calculation for Aromatic (benzoyl system) compounds

λ max = Basic value + Substitution effect (ortho or meta or para)

Basic values:

- (a) Ar-COR (ketone)   =   246 nm
- (b) Ar-CHO (Aldehyde)   =   250 nm
- (c) Ar-CO₂H (Acid)   =   230 nm
- (d) Ar-CO₂R (Ester)   =   230 nm

Value (in nm) for Substitution effect (ortho or meta or para)

Table 1.6 λ max for structural futures

Auxochrome	ortho	meta	para
-NR2 (amine)	20	20	85
-NH2	13	13	58
-NHCH3	-	-	73
-NHCOCH3	20	20	45
-OH , -OR	7	7	25
Alipahtic (- R)	3	3	10
-Br	2	2	15
-Cl	0	0	10
-O+ (oxonium)	11	20	78

Example:

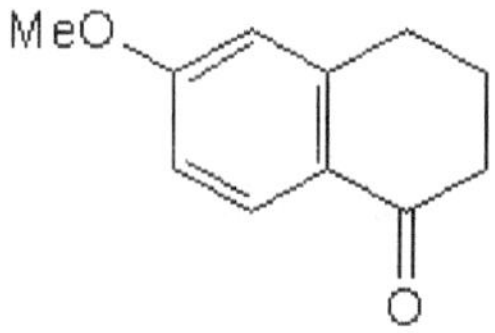

λ max = 230 nm (base value) + 58 nm (-NH2 at para position)

= 288 nm

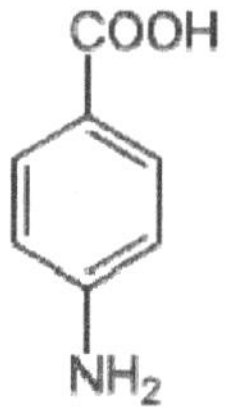

λ max = 246 nm (base value) + 3 nm (alkyl ring residue) + 25 nm (OCH3 at para position)

= 274 nm

Exercise: *calculate the □ max for the following structure ?*

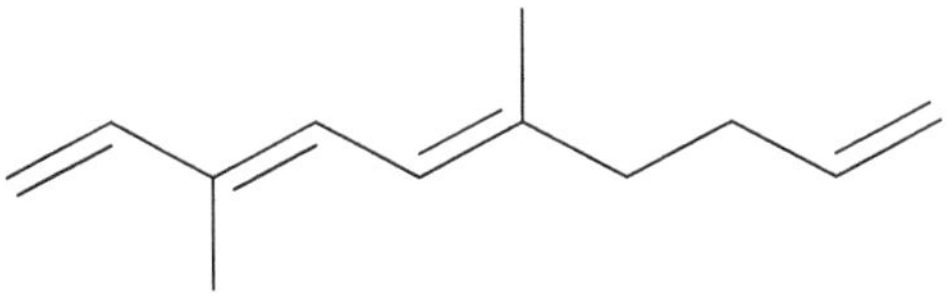

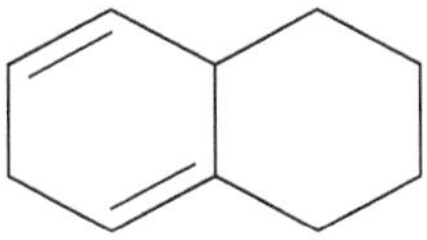

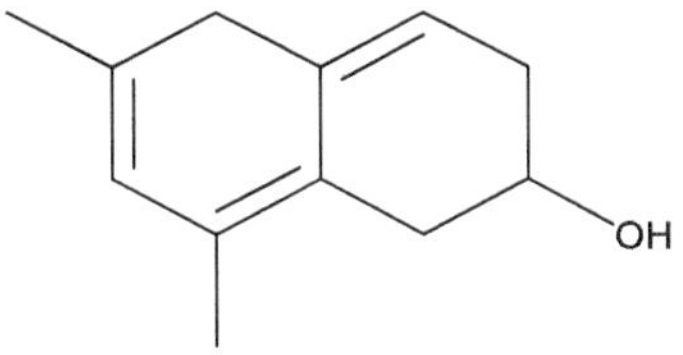

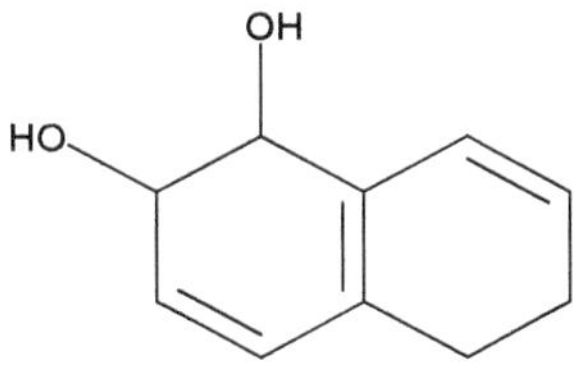

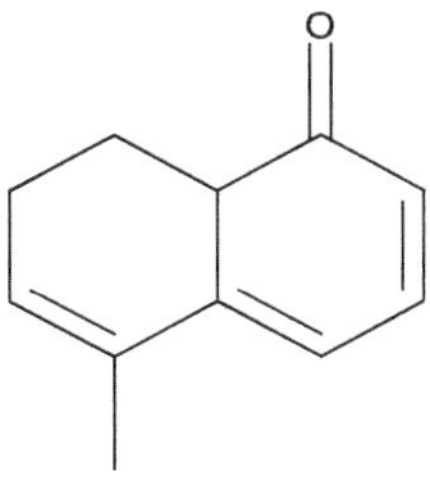

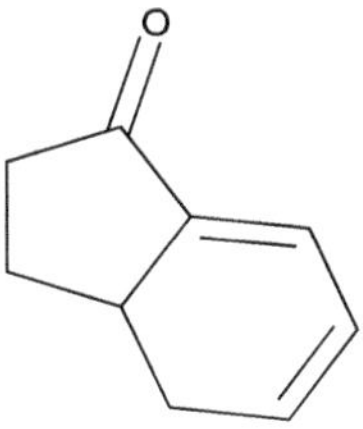

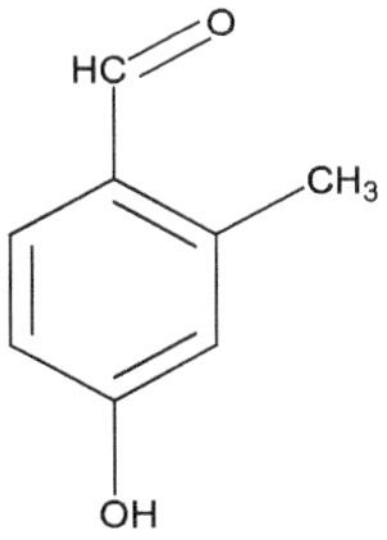

Chapter 2

Infra Red (IR) Spectroscopy

Infrared spectroscopy (IR spectroscopy) is a type of absorption spectroscopy based on absorption of infrared region (IR radiation) of the electromagnetic spectrum (light with a longer wavelength and lower energy than visible light) by the vibrating bonds in the molecule. It can represent the identify of chemical structure based on functional groups, Bonds, isomerism (except optical isomerism) study chemicals. For a given sample which may be solid, liquid, or gaseous, with suitable sample technique and with the use of **infrared spectrometer** (or spectrophotometer), the **infrared (IR) spectrum can be obtained**. A basic IR spectrum is essentially a graph based on infrared light absorbance (or transmittance) on the vertical Y-axis vs. frequency (Hz) or wavelength (micron) or wavenumber (Cm-1) on the horizontal X-axis. More commonly a unit of frequency used wavenumber (reciprocal centimeters of wavelength) is used in interpretation of spectra. A common laboratory instrument in present day is a Fourier transform infrared (FTIR) spectrometer.

Table 2.1 Different units and regions of IR radiation and their effect on organic molecules

Region	Frequency	Effect on molecule
Near IR	14000–4000 cm^{-1} (0.8–2.5 µm)	The higher-energy near-IR, approximately can excite overtone or harmonic vibrations
Middle IR	4000–400 cm^{-1} (2.5–25 µm)	The mid-infrared, approximately may be used to study the fundamental vibrations and associated rotational-vibrational structure. (organic and pharmaceuticals)
Far IR	400–10 cm^{-1} (25–1000 µm),	The far-infrared, approximately lying adjacent to the microwave region, has low energy and may be used for rotational spectroscopy

Molecular Vibration and IR Absorption

Every bond in the molecule is under vibration, due to variety reason if m1 and m2 are mass of the atom and K is the force constant, the vibration of bond can be calculated using Hooke's law

Fundamental frequency of the bond (natural) =

$$\bar{v} = \frac{1}{2x} \sqrt{\frac{k}{\mu}} \qquad \mu = \frac{m_1 \cdot m_2}{m_1 + m_2}$$

$\bar{v}$ = frequency μ = reduced mass

NOTE: *For a molecule to be "IR active (absorbs IR radiation), it must be associated with changes in the dipole, remember that permanent dipole is not necessary, but requires only a change in dipole moment.*

A molecule can vibrate in several ways (called *vibrational mode*). If N' number of atoms in a linear molecules have $3N - 5$ degrees of vibrational modes, whereas nonlinear molecules have $3N - 6$ degrees of vibrational modes (also called vibrational degrees of freedom).

As an example H_2O, a non-linear molecule, will have $3 \times 3 - 6 = 3$ degrees of vibrational freedom, or modes.

NOTE: *Simple diatomic molecules have only one bond and only one vibrational band. If the molecule is symmetrical, e.g. N_2, the band is not observed in the IR spectrum but only in the Raman spectrum. Asymmetrical diatomic molecules, e.g. CO, absorb in the IR spectrum. More complex molecules have many bonds, and their vibrational spectra are correspondingly more complex, i.e. big molecules have many peaks in their IR spectra'.*

The-CH_2-group is more commonly found in organic compounds, can vibrate in different ways. Six of these vibrations are **symmetric and antisymmetric stretching, scissoring, rocking, wagging** and **twisting,** as shown in Figure 2.1A (*The rocking, wagging, and twisting modes do not exist for H_2O, since they are rigid body translations and no relative displacements exist*)

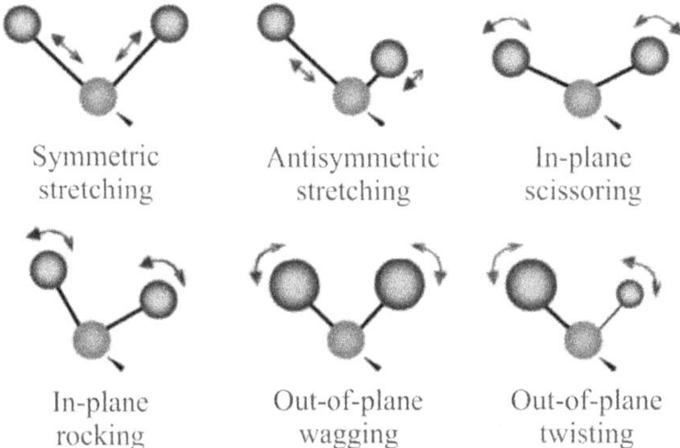

Figure 2.1A Types of vibrations in an organic molecules.

The irradiated IR radiation is absorbed by the bond when fundamental frequency is equal to the applied IR frequency, as a result the change vibration energy takes place (V0 to V1). A typical representation of IR absorption for C=O group of 2 – hexanone is shown in Figure 2.1B. Same applicable for other bond in the molecule.

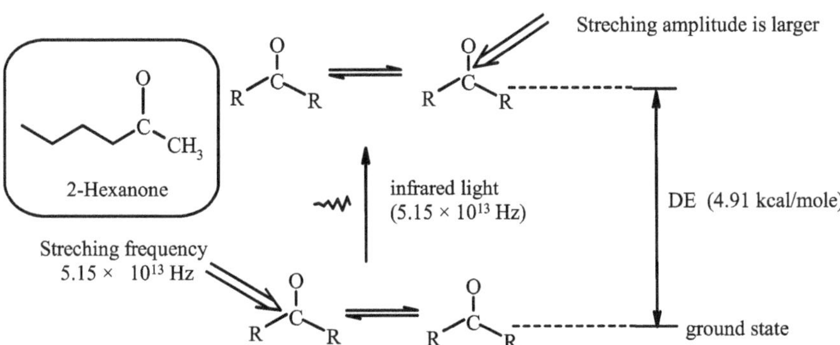

Figure 2.1B Typical IR radiation absorption by C=O (carbonyl group) in a molecule.

Hence all bond as well as all modes of vibration possess different fundamental frequency, different bond absorbs different frequency. The fundamental region for different bonds in organic molecules is shown below (Figure 2.1C).

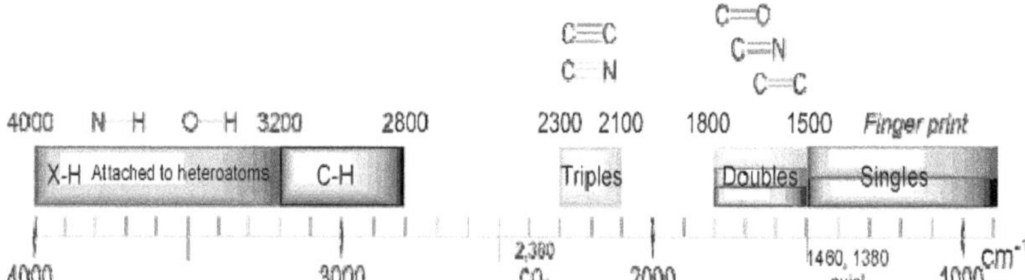

Figure 2.1C Different IR regions and its corresponding vibrational frequency of bond.

It also noted that for a same bond or functional group, the IR absorption frequency is different for different mode.

Interpretation of FT – IR Spectrum for Functional Groups

The interpretation of infrared spectra involves the correlation of absorption bands in the spectrum of an unknown compound with the known absorption frequencies for types of bonds (functional groups). The following table will help us to identify the functional groups based on absorption band position (with frequencies in wavenumber cm-1). Significant for the identification of the source of an absorption band are **intensity** (weak, medium or strong), **shape** (broad or sharp), and **position** (cm⁻¹) in the spectrum.

There two different region: Group frequency region (4000-1100 cm-1) and finger print region (1100-400 cm-1). Finger print region is very sensitive for small change in the structure, so it can be used for identification and authentication.

Table 2.2 Characteristic middle infra-red (MIR) absorption frequencies for various chemical compounds

Bond	Compound Type	Frequency range, cm⁻¹
C-H	Alkanes	2960-2850(s) stretch
		1470-1350(v) scissoring and bending
	CH₃ Umbrella Deformation	1380(m-w) - Doublet - isopropyl, *t*-butyl
C-H	Alkenes	3080-3020(m) stretch
		1000-675(s) bend
C-H	Aromatic Rings	3100-3000(m) stretch
	Phenyl Ring Substitution Bands	870-675(s) bend
	Phenyl Ring Substitution Overtones	2000-1600(w) - fingerprint region

Table 2.2 contd...

Bond	Compound Type	Frequency range, cm⁻¹
C-H	Alkynes	3333-3267(s) stretch
		700-610(b) bend
C=C	Alkenes	1680-1640(m,w)) stretch
C≡C	Alkynes	2260-2100(w,sh) stretch
C=C, C=N	Aromatic Rings	1600, 1500(w) stretch
C-O	Alcohols, Ethers, Carboxylic acids, Esters	1260-1000(s) stretch
C=O	Aldehydes, Ketones, Carboxylic acids, Esters	1760-1670(s) stretch
O-H	Monomeric -- Alcohols, Phenols	3640-3160(s,br) stretch
	Hydrogen-bonded – Alcohols, Phenols	3600-3200(b) stretch
	Carboxylic acids	3000-2500(b) stretch
N-H	Amines	3500-3300(m) stretch
		1650-1580 (m) bend
C-N	Amines	1340-1020(m) stretch
C≡N	Nitriles	2260-2220(v) stretch
NO₂	Nitro Compounds	1660-1500(s) asymmetrical stretch
		1390-1260(s) symmetrical stretch

v - Variable, m - medium, s - strong, br - broad, w - weak

Example Interpretation of Infrared Spectra

Illustrated example 1:

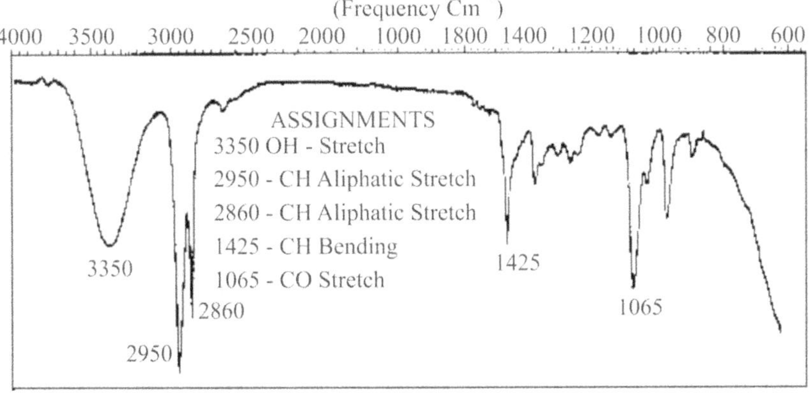

Figure 2.2 Interpretation of IR spectra for various functional groups

The above unknown spectrum represents the presence of OH, CH, C-O group in the structure.

Illustrated example 2:

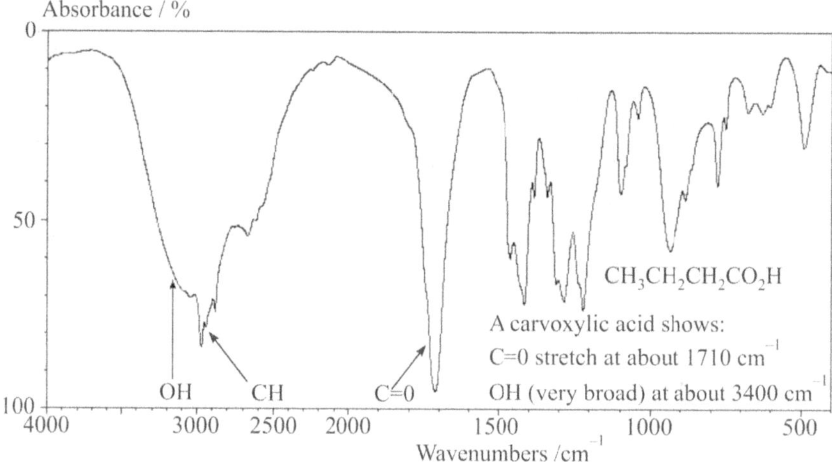

Figure 2.3 IR spectra of Botanic acid.

Illustrated example 3:

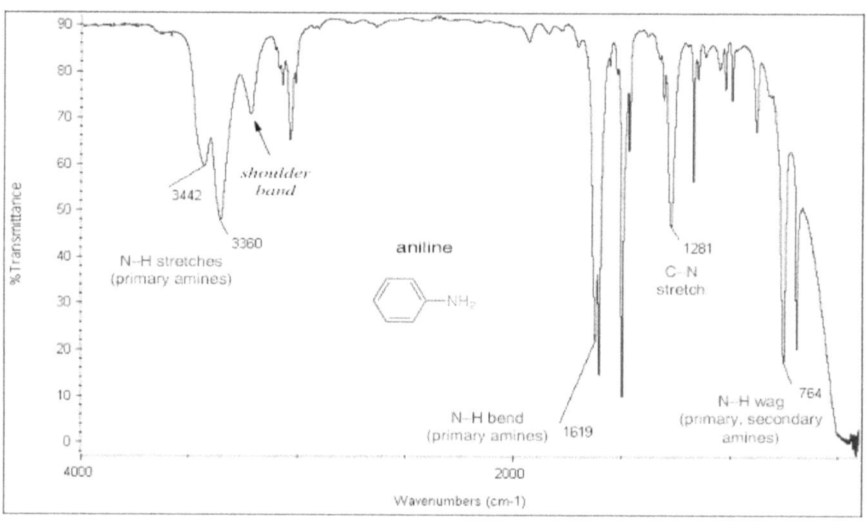

Figure 2.4 IR spectra of Aniline.

Perform interpretation for the following Spectrum using the above table?

Example 1:

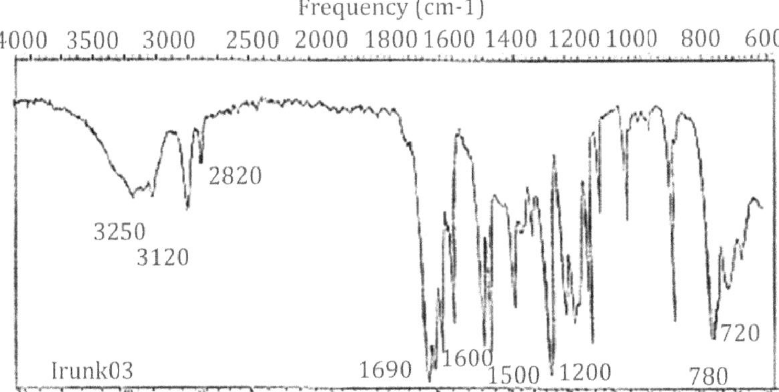

Figure 2.5 IR spectra.

Example 2:

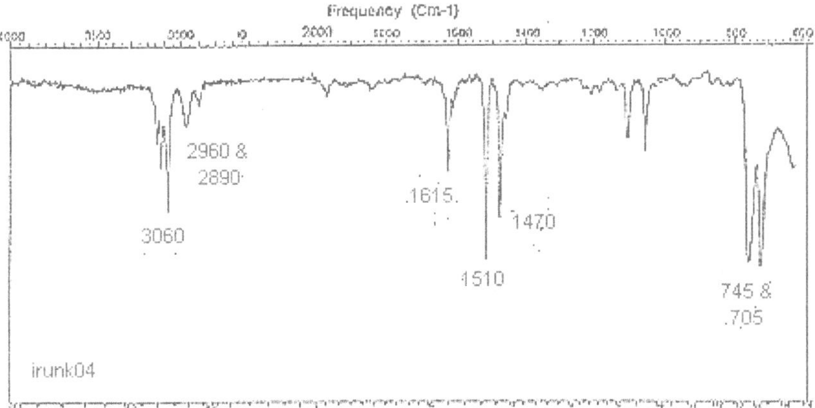

Figure 2.6 Unknown IR spectra.

Example 3:

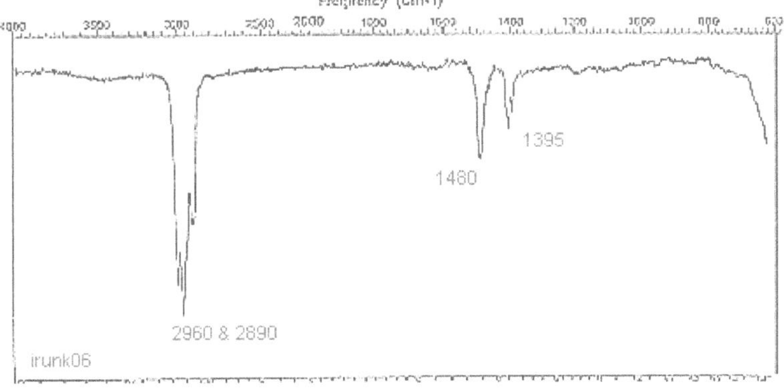

Figure 2.7 Unknown IR spectra.

Identification of Optimum Spectra for Studies

The resolution of IR spectra depends on the amount of sample, suitable sample technique and instrument sensitivity. The following spectra (Figure 2.8) shows the effect of sample concentration on IR spectra.

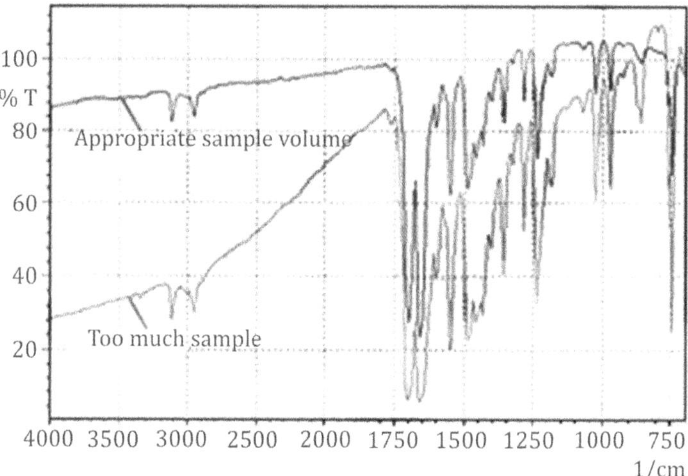

Figure 2.8 Comparative IR spectra of different sample amount in KBr pellet.

Identification of Hydrogen bonding in IR Spectrum

The hydrogen bonding of OH is more observed as very broad band over the region between 3200-3600 cm-1. Free OH band appears as intense and sharp. But hydrogen bonded OH appears as broad band. In Figure 2.9, the shaded region shows the hydrogen bonds. In Figure 2.10, the broad absorption at 3400 cm-1 shows hydrogen bonded–OH bond vibrations of 2-propanol.

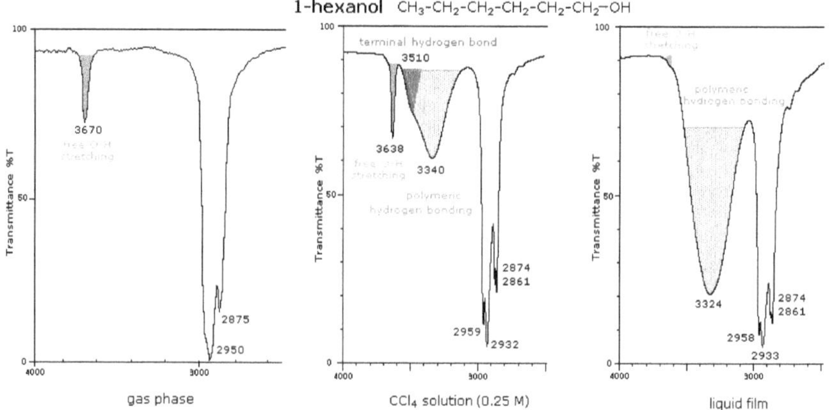

Figure 2.9 IR spectra of 1-hexanol in different Phase (Focus on H-bonding).

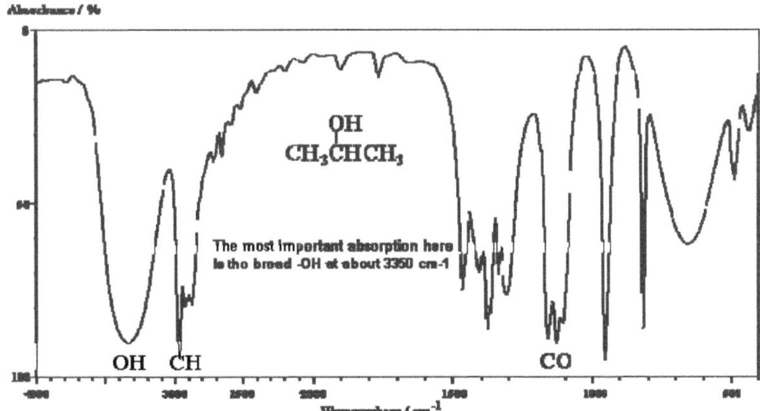

Figure 2.10 IR spectra of 2-propanol.

Identification / authentication of Compounds by Fingerprint matching:

Identification pharmaceuticals are more commonly recommended by many Pharmacopoeias, like IP, BP, and USP-NF. It involves the process of overlap the standard and Test spectrum and examine for the matching of absorption pattern. It is more commonly done in between 2000-400 cm-1. The following spectrum (Figure 2.11) shows the example of identification of four samples of same chemical nature.

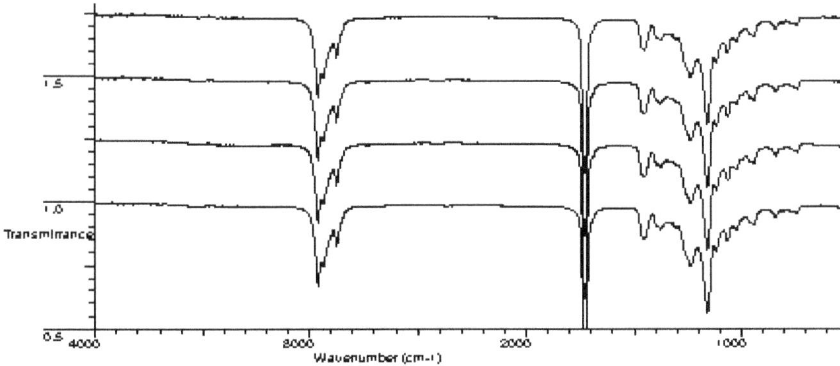

Figure 2.11 Fingerprint matching IR spectra sample of different production batch.

Differentiation of Positional Isomers

The finger print regions (1100 – 400 cm-1) will be highly preferred for differentiation of positional isomers, for example 1- propanol and 2 –

propanol has different absorption pattern in fingerprint region as shown in Figure 2.12

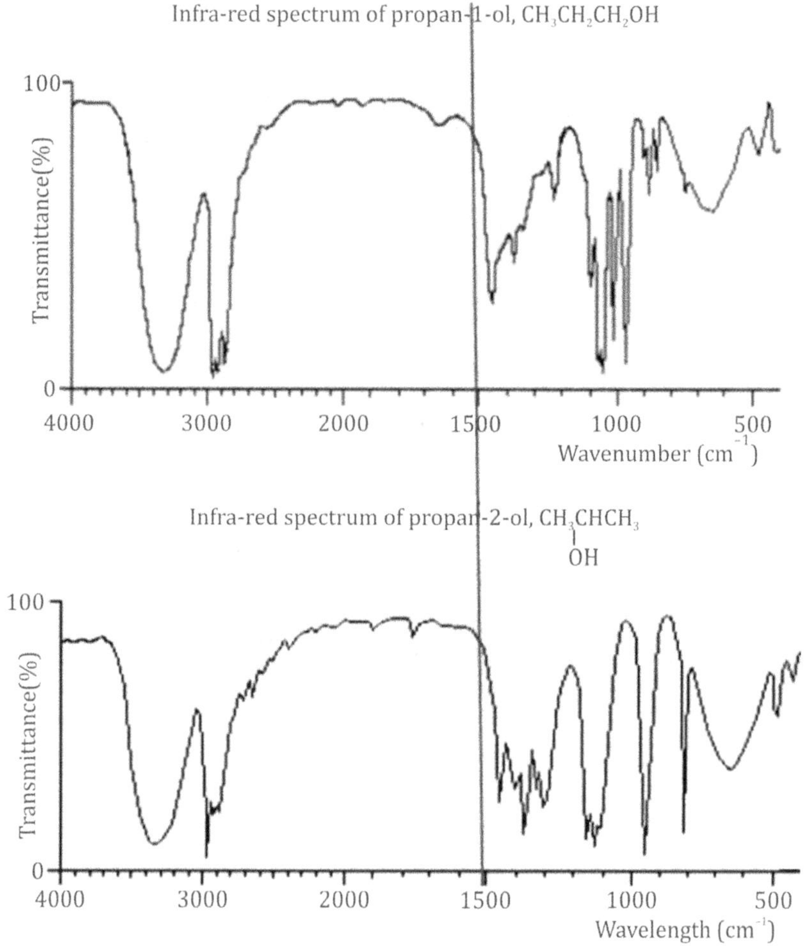

Figure 2.12 IR spectra of Propan-1-ol and Propan-2-ol.

Detection of Impurity in Pharmaceuticals

The following reaction shows the chemical reaction for the synthesis of paracetamol. There prominent impurity may be Para- aminophenol di-acetylated by product.

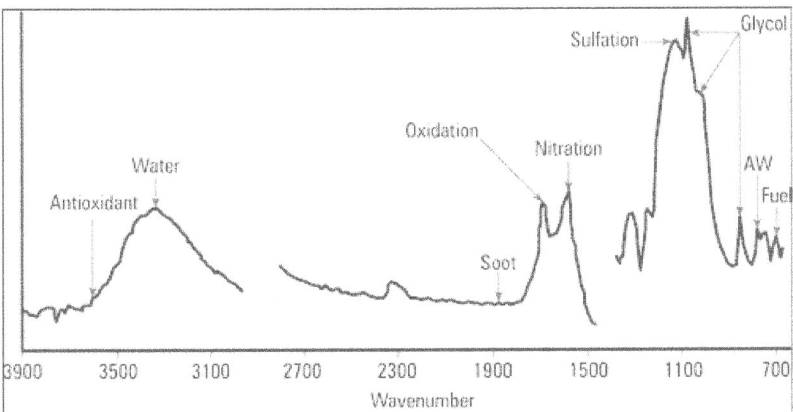

The important functional groups represent impurity is – NH2 group (around 3300 cm-1). The following spectrum (Figure 2.13) shows the IR absorption characteristics of denatured oil.

Figure 2.13 IR spectrum of denatured oil (absorption mode of IR spectrum).

The following overlay spectrum (Figure 2.14) shows the presence of band at 3394 and 1706 indicated the presence of used (oxidized) oil. The decision can be made in comparison with pure (fresh) oil.

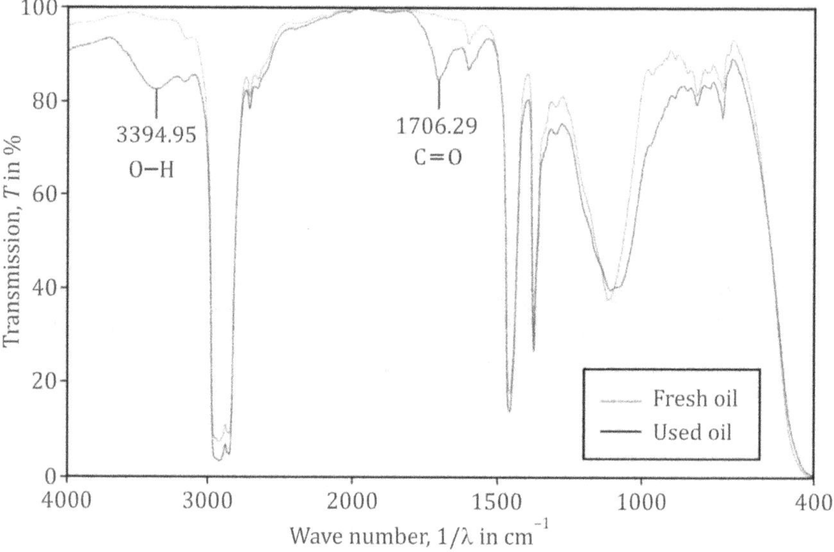

Figure 2.14 IR spectra of oxidized oil Vs Fresh oil.

Detection of Chemical Compatibility of Ibuprofen by IR

The identification and detection of pharmaceuticals in dosage form can be done using comparison among excipients, pure drug and dosage form spectra. The chemical compatibility should not be assessed without placebo (only excipients) and standard drug spectra.

The following spectrum (Figure 2.15) shows the chemical compatibility and identification of ibuprofen in the tablet dosage form.

- The interpretation made based on the presence of characteristics functional groups in formulation.

- Check for presence of new or absence of characteristic bands while comparing the formulation with placebo and pure drugs.

- Check for drastic shift of band to higher or lower frequency, due to complex formation. The shift around 2-4 cm^{-1} should not be considered as interaction.

- Some time the formulation is based on the complex formation, it could be noticed the drastic shift of bands and change in intensity of absorption.

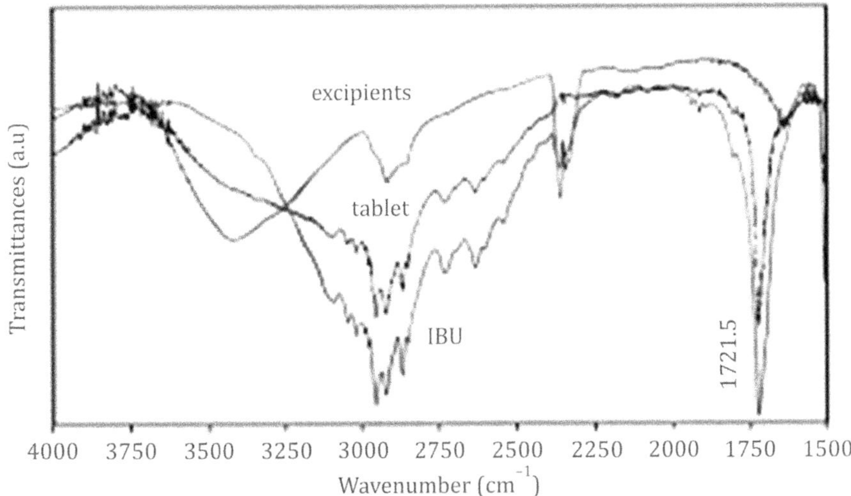

Figure 2.15 IR spectra of chemical compatibility and identification of Ibuprofen.

The following spectrum (Figure 2.16) indicates the compatibility of diltiazem hydrochloride.

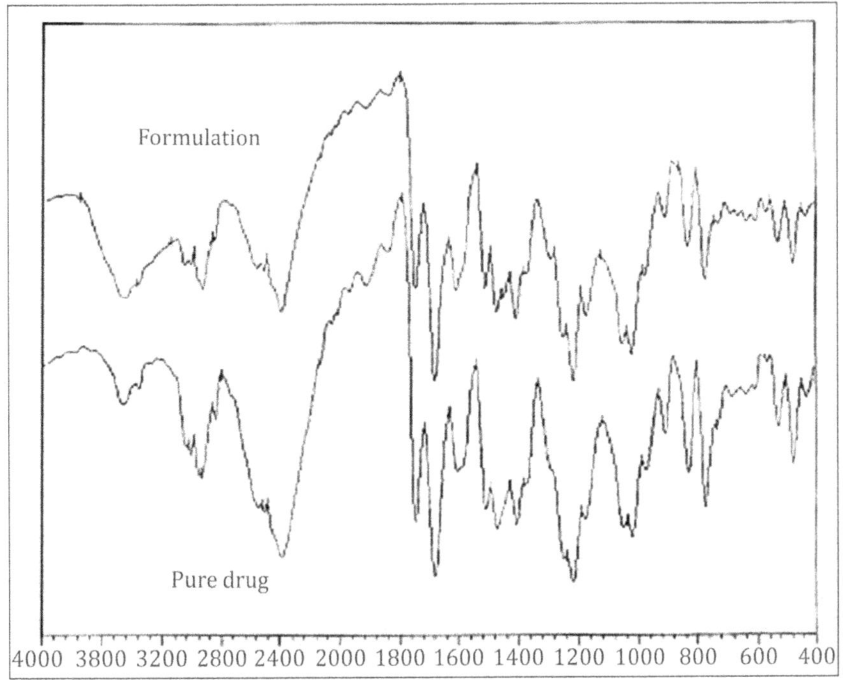

Figure 2.16 IR spectrum of diltiazem hydrochloride.

Detection of Polymorphism

NOTE: Do not use KBr pellet technique and solution phase to study Polymorphism, choose ATR or DRS technique for polymorphism.

IR spectra (Figure 2.14) of three forms of the co-crystal system, 4-hydroxybenzoic acid: 4,4′-bipyridine (2 : 1), show clear differences that may be attributed to differences in the synthon combinations existing in the forms (synthon polymorphism).

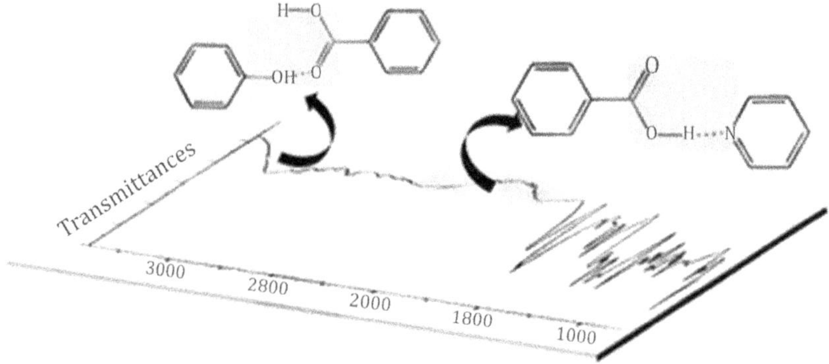

Figure 2.17 IR spectrum of 4-hydroxybenzoic acid: 4,4′-bipyridine.

The following spectrum (Figure 2.18) shows the difference in the OH interaction in different polymorph (Form1, Form2, and Form3)

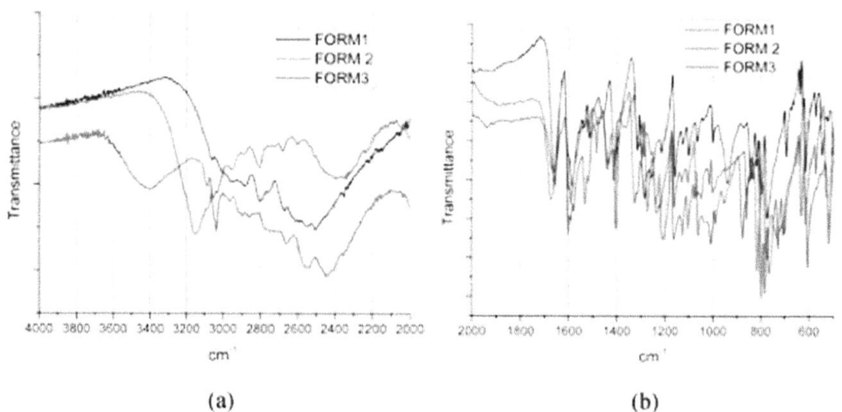

Figure 2.18 IR spectra of OH interaction in different polymorph.

NOTE: In addition to IR, it is always recommended to study the polymorph by Raman Spectra (absorption mode). From the following figure 2.19 we can observe that different forms of carbamazepine have different absorption pattern.

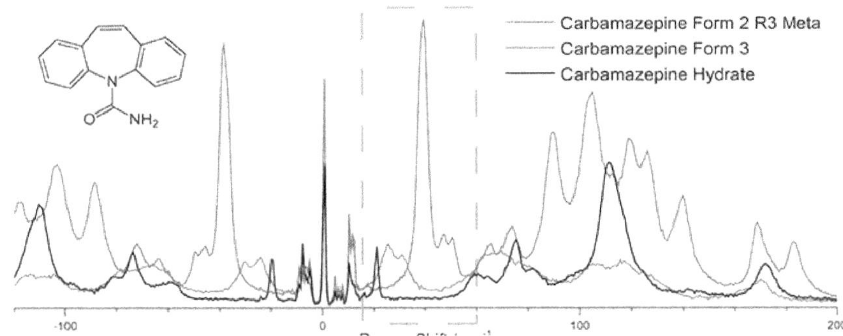

Figure 2.19 IR spectra of carbamazepine polymorphs.

Detection of Bio-molecules in Serum/Biological Samples

The following table gives the information of rat serum and human serum by IR spectroscopy. Overline IR-ATR spectra (Figure 2.20) (a) Disease control; (b) metformin treated (1 h); and (c)normal control Intensity Ration Parameters (IRP) values can be used to study the levels of different biochemical levels (but not accurately). Table 2.3 shows the IR absorption regions for biomolecules.

ATR Techniques: ATR (attenuated total reflection) is a technique for obtaining IR spectra of samples that are difficult to deal with, such as solids of limited solubility, films, threads, pastes, adhesives, and powders. In this process, a beam of radiation entering a crystal will undergo total internal reflection when the angle of incidence at the interface between the sample and the crystal is greater than the critical angle. The critical angle is a function of the refractive indices of the two surfaces. The beam penetrates a fraction of a wavelength beyond the reflecting surface and when a material that selectively absorbs radiation is in close contact with the reflecting surface, the beam loses energy at the wavelength where the material absorbs. The resultant attenuated radiation is measured and plotted as a function of the wavelength by the spectrometer and gives rise to the absorption spectral characteristics of the sample.

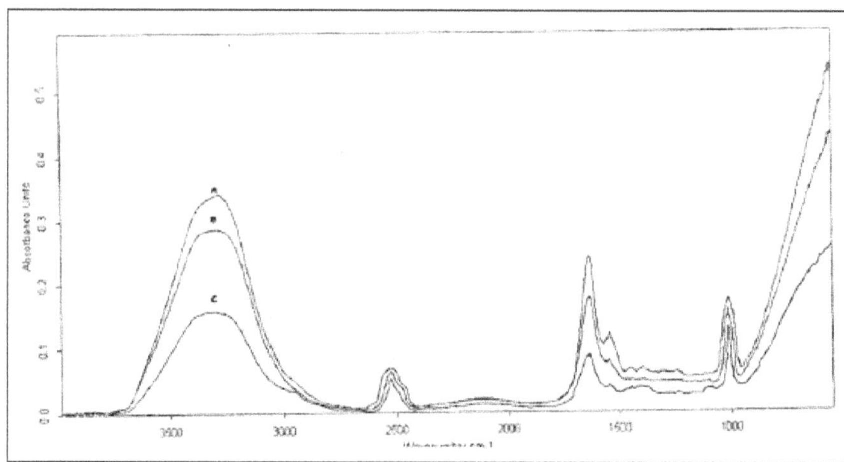

Figure 2.20 IR spectrum of absorption characteristics of biological samples.

Table 2.3 Detection of biomolecules in serum/biological samples

Rat serum		Human serum	
Frequency (cm^{-1})	Assignments	Frequency (cm^{-1})	Assignments
702	N–H out of plane deformation of protein	702	N–H out of plane deformation of protein
1018	C–O stretch of β-anomer	1035	C–O stretch of β-anomer
1079	C–O stretch of α-anomer	1079	C–O stretch of α-anomer
1109	Endocyclic C–O–C vibration	1107	Endocyclic C–O–C vibration
1153	Ring vibration modes of C–O–C and C–O–H bonds	1153	Ring vibration modes of C–O–C and C–O–H bonds
1169	C–O stretch of COH tyrosine protein	1169	C–O stretch of COH tyrosine protein
1315	CH$_2$ vibrations of α-anomer	1315	CH$_2$ vibrations of α-anomer
1365	CH$_2$ vibrations of β-anomer	1365	CH$_2$ vibrations of β-anomer
1400	CH$_3$ symmetric bending vibration of protein	1400	CH$_3$ symmetric bending vibration of protein
1435	C–H bending	1435	C–H bending
1456	CH$_3$ asymmetric bending vibration of protein	1456	CH$_3$ asymmetric bending vibration of protein
1645	C=O stretching/C–N stretching/N–H bending of proteins (amide I band)	1655	C=O stretching/C–N stretching/N–H bending of proteins (amide I band)
1551	N–H bending strongly coupled with C–N stretching (amide II band)	1548	N–H bending strongly coupled with C–N stretching (amide II band)
2846	CH$_2$ symmetric stretching	2851	CH$_2$ symmetric stretching
2871	CH$_2$ asymmetric stretching	2871	CH$_2$ asymmetric stretching
2922	CH$_3$ symmetric stretching of proteins and lipids	2922	CH$_3$ symmetric stretching of proteins and lipids
2961	CH$_3$ asymmetric stretching of proteins and lipids	2956	CH$_3$ asymmetric stretching of proteins and lipids
3366	N–H asymmetric stretching of secondary amides of proteins	3400	N–H asymmetric stretching of secondary amides of proteins

Differentiation of Geometric Isomers

Infrared spectra provide are one of the tool for differentiating isomeric organic compounds. The restricted rotation about C=C, will have significant impact in absorption pattern of C=C and other bonds in the molecule.

NOTE: Finger print region in IR spectroscopy is to be used in the determination of E-Z compounds. 970–960 for trans-C-H out-of-plane bends; whereas 700 (broad) cis-C-H out-of-planebend. FTIR allow unambiguous determination of the configuration of the double bonds in long chain unsaturated compounds bearing a RCH=CHR' types of bonds (Figure 2.21).

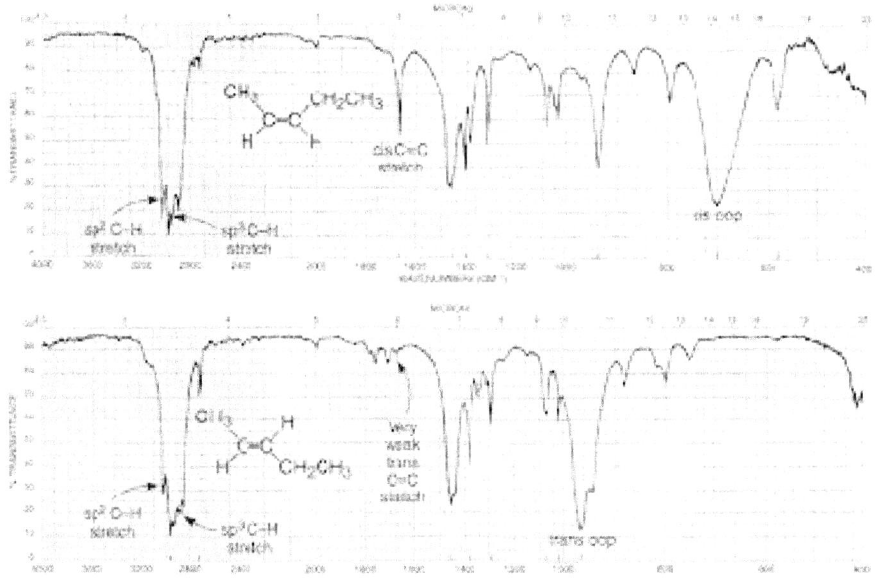

Figure 2.21 IR spectrum of Geometric isomers.

Example: (α-asarone) and β-asarone (**II** and **I**). The IR spectrum (Figure 2.22) of both form will have different absorption pattern in between 1400-800 cm-1

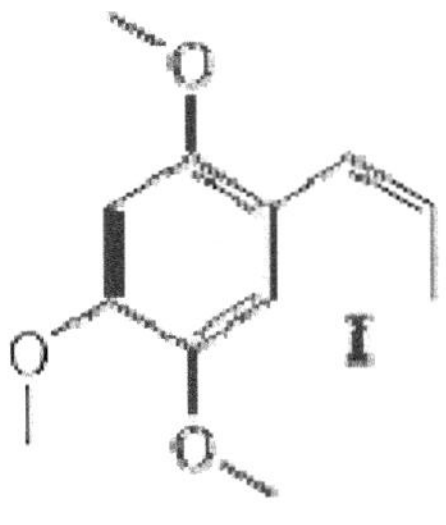

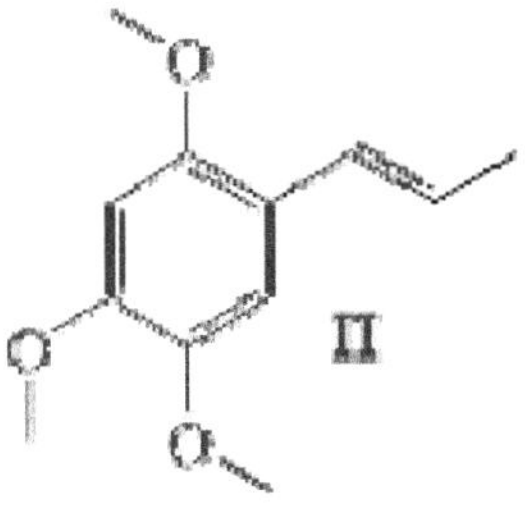

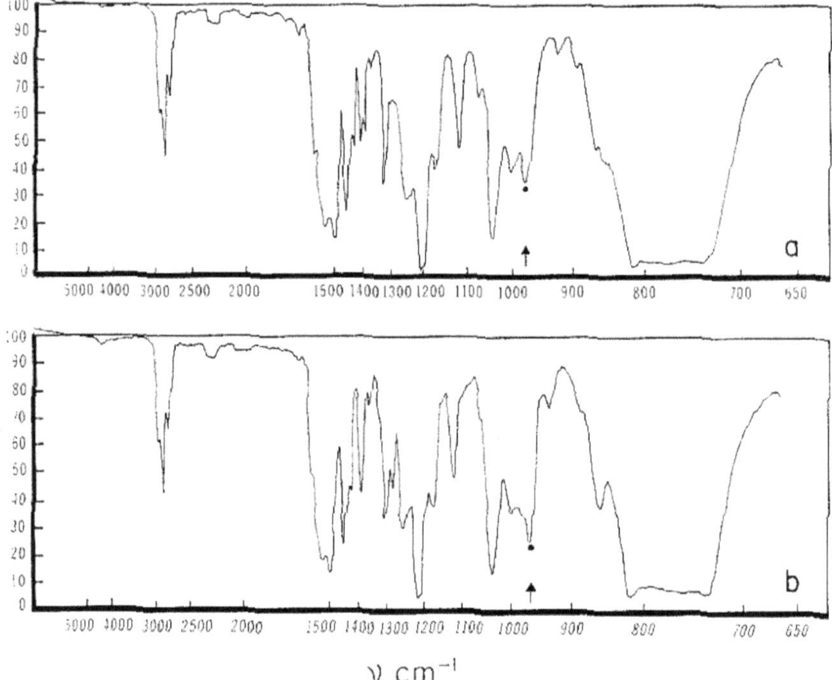

Figure 2.22 IR spectrum of α-asarone and β-asarone.

Differentiation of Aromatic Positional Isomers

Many of characterized IR bands show the substitution pattern on aromatic rings. As an example, the C-H wagging band near 800 cm-1 differentiates between ortho (~750), meta (~770),and para (~805) isomers, as shown in the Figure 2.23.

For example Xylene,

From the following figure we can observe that the absorption frequency for out-of-plane is lowest for para, among all. The order of frequency is para< meta< ortho.

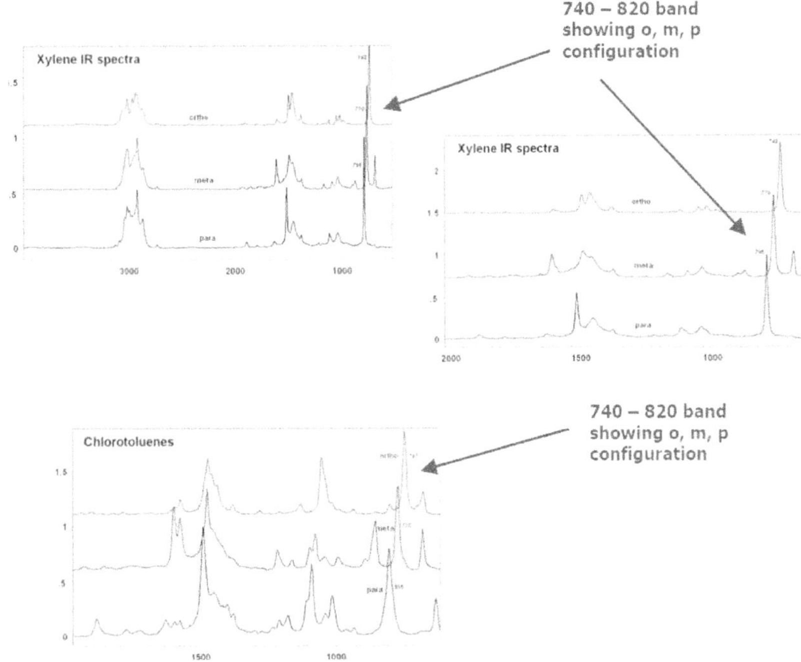

Figure 2.23 IR spectra of aromatic positional isomers.

IR Finger Prints for Herbal Drug Standardization

Now a day, IR spectrum of extract, of pure chemical components is used as standard to detect the standard of crude drugs and their products. The following IR spectra (Figure 2.24) show the Finger print of all major components in clove oil, which can be used to identify the unknown sample.

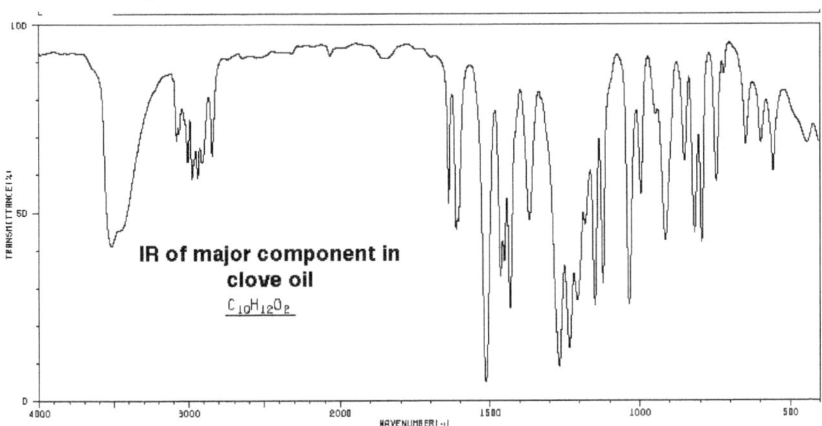

Figure 2.24 IR spectrum of clove oil.

Example: The following figure 2.25 shows the comparison of tea and its infusion to assess the standards of decomposition during infusion. Since, spectra are superimposable at all frequencies, it can be concluded the identity and stability

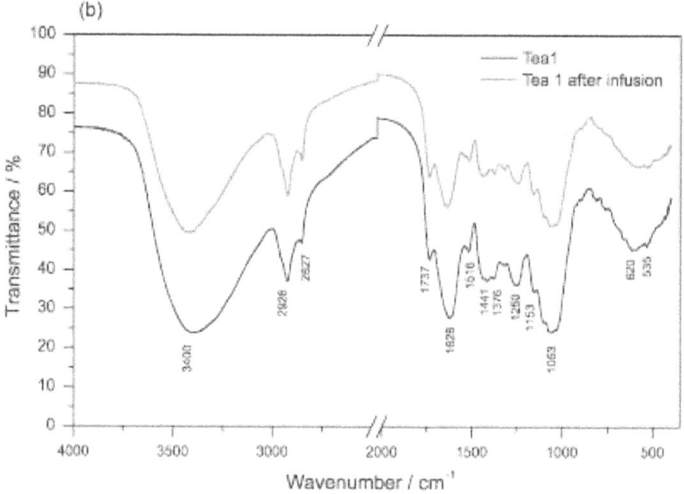

Figure 2.25 IR spectrum of tea.

Authentication of drug products: The following spectrum (Figure 2.26) shows the authentication fungal extracted Taxol (a) with standard Taxol (b).

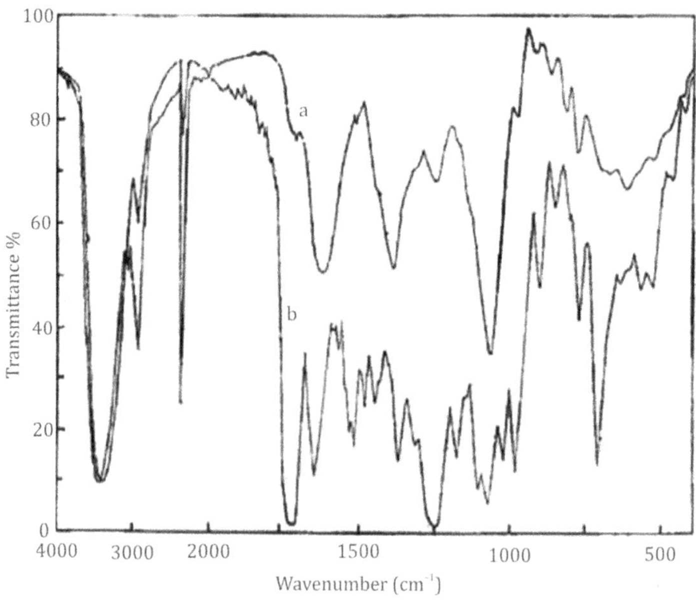

Figure 2.26 IR spectra of taxol (a) with standard taxol (b).

Quantification by IR Spectroscopy using Baseline Technique

Similar to that of UV-spectroscopy, based on beers law the intensity of the absorption for a particular characteristic band (example: C=O, C=N) can be measured, using baseline correction to 100 % or with adjustment. The following Figure 2.27 shows the absorbance measurement using the transmittance compound for a particular band (P_0) and transmittance at baseline (P_B).

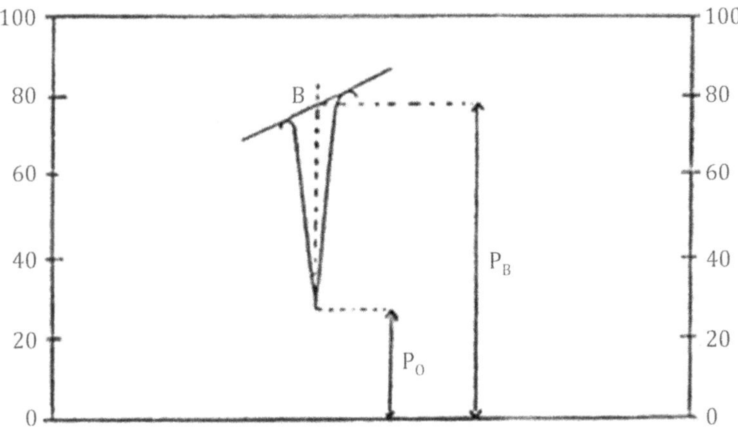

Figure 2.27 IR spectroscopy using baseline technique.

The Absorbance = Transmittance of P_B - Transmittance of P_0

Studying the Progress of the Reaction

Progress of a chemical reaction can be determined by examining the small portion of the reaction mixture withdrawn from time to time. The rate of disappearance of a characteristic absorption band of the reactant group and/or the rate of appearance of the characteristic absorption band of the product group due to formation of product is observed.

Example: Figure 2.28 shows the Conversion of benzene (a) to trinitrobenzene (NO2) group (b), then reduction to amino-benzene (c) (NH2)

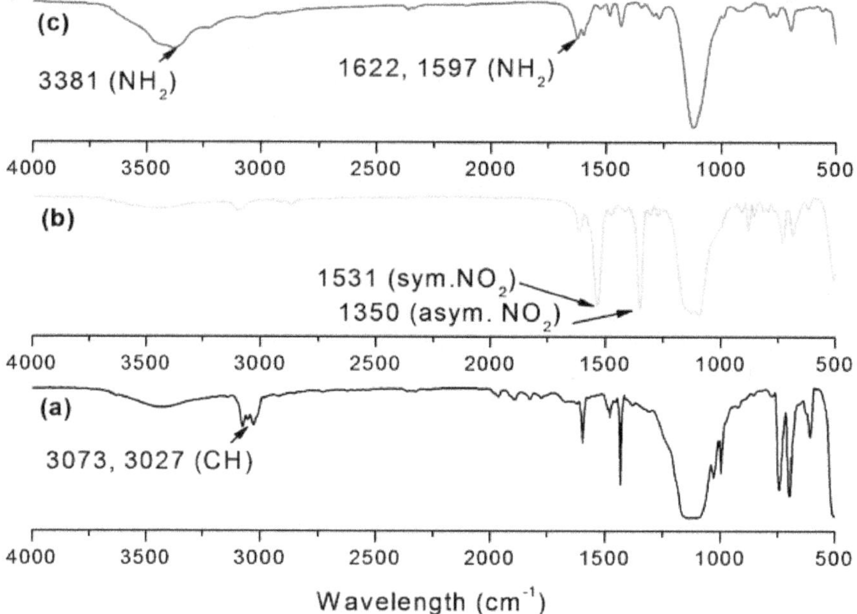

Figure 2.28 IR spectra of (a) benzene (b) tri-nitrobenzene (c) amino-benzene.

Detection of Degradation

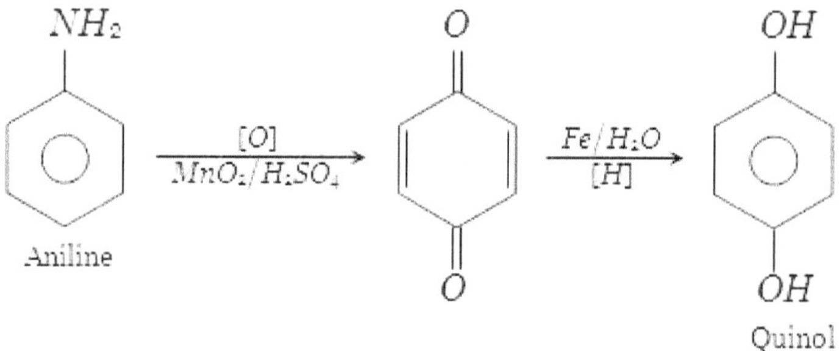

Figure 2.29 Scheme of aniline degradation to quinol.

When aniline oxidized, it produce Quinone and quinol. The difference in the functional group between aniline and its degradation products can be done by IR Spectra (Figure 2.29).

Chapter 3

H⁻¹ NMR Spectroscopy

Proton NMR (also **Hydrogen-1 NMR** or 1 H **NMR**) is a type of nuclear magnetic resonance in NMR spectroscopy represents the hydrogen (H^1 isotope - Proton) within the molecules of a substance, in order to determine the structure of its molecules. In samples 99.99 % will be proton isotope rest will be deuterium and tritium.

NMR spectroscopy is based on the absorption of radiofrequency (rf) by the spinning nuclei (Spin quantum number I > 0, if I = 0 indicate the nuclei does not possess spin, hence they do not absorb radiofrequency). In general if atomic number and weight are even the spin quantum number become zero (Example C12 do not absorb radio frequency but C13 absorbs radiofrequency.

Principle of Radiofrequency Absorption

Any spinning nuclei (I > 0) will have different energy level under external field, and the number of energy level is depends on spin quantum number. For example both H1 and C13 nuclei possess spin quantum number of half integral (I = ½), where H2 possess integral (I = 1).

Hence the number of energy level for C13 and H1 will be based on the formula (2I + 1), hence two energy level +1/2 and -1/2 respectively for higher energy (bête) and lower energy (alpha) orientations with the applied magnetic field. But remember the spin direction is opposite but the frequency will be same.

Hence for the given nuclei, the spinning frequency of the proton or C13 under magnetic field is calculated from the following frequency.

$$\nu = \frac{\gamma B_o}{2\pi} \quad \text{for } {}^{1}\text{H, } \nu \text{ is 60 MHz for } B_o = 14.092 \text{ gauss}$$

$$\gamma = \text{magnetogyric ratio} = 26.753 \text{ radians/gauss for } {}^{1}\text{H}$$

$$\gamma = \frac{2\pi\mu}{hI} \quad \mu = \text{magnetic moment}$$

Hence the Larmor frequency (Precessional frequency) is depends on the applied magnetic field and has be depends on the radio frequency used. The excitation process is shown in Figure 3.1.

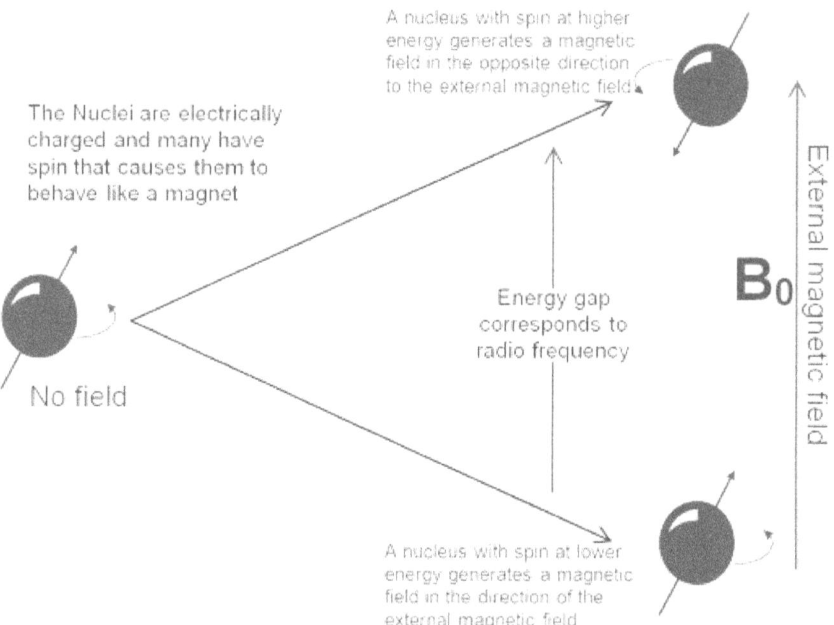

Figure 3.1 Excitation (Flipping) process of Nuclei in NMR spectroscopy due radiofrequency.

The radiofrequency used will be 60, 90, 100, 300, 600 MHz, as the frequency increases, the resolution increases. Radiofrequency is absorbed by a molecule only when,

Precessional Frequency (Larmor) = Applied radiofrequency (Rf)

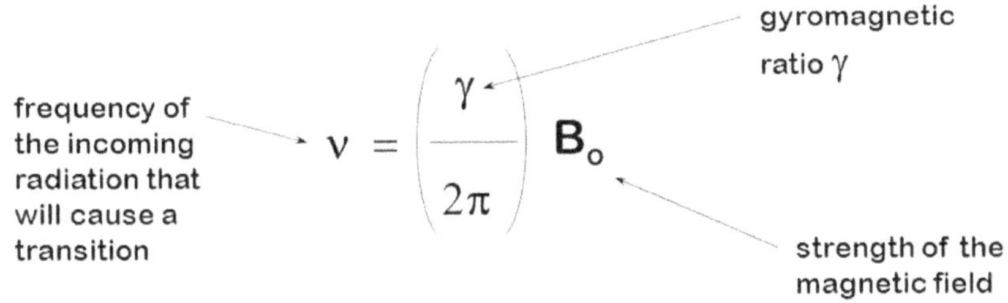

The above equation is called LARMOR equation represent the Fundamental NMR equation.

Where gyromagnetic ratio differ from nuclei to nuclei and depending on the environments. During instrumentation, the magnetic sweep is followed where the applied frequency kept constant, the mangetic scan is performed. Hence, the NMR spectrum is recorded, based on the applied magnetic energy in X axis and Rf absorbance in Y-axis. At applied magnetic frequency, no two protons will have same precessional energy unless they are magnetically equivalent. The instrumentation is shown in Figure 3.2.

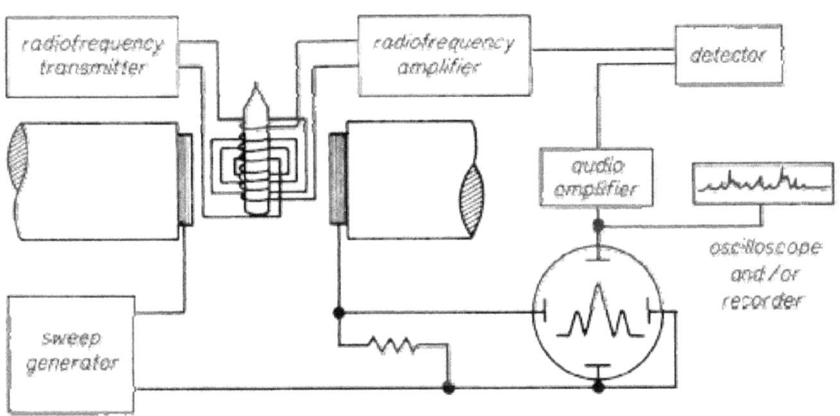

Figure 3.2 NMR spectrophotometer.

Example: CH3OH – Environment of CH3 proton and OH proton are different (Figure 3.4). Hence they are magnetically not equivalent and absorb different energy and give different signal.

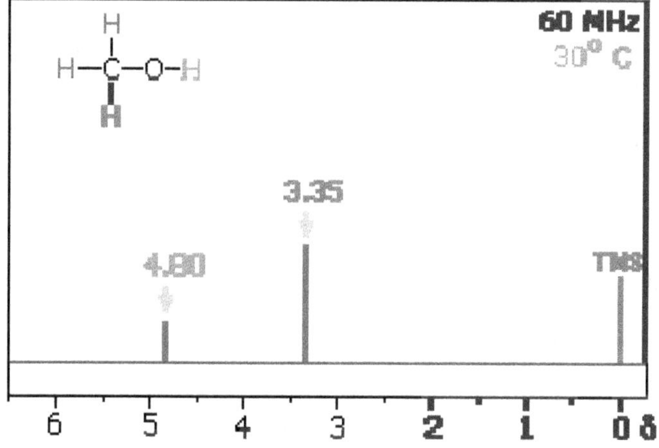

Figure 3.3 NMR spectrum of Methanol.

Same way example of Ethanol: Which has three type of proton, CH3, CH2, OH absorb different frequency (figure 3.4). In NMR spectrum, signal at 0 ppm, is due to internal standard (tetramethylsilane so called TMS, which is used for calibration of chemical shift scale). The TMS give once signal, because all four CH3 group are attached to one Silicon atom, and considered as all 12 protons 4 CH3) are magnetically equivalent.

$$CH_3$$
$$H_3C-Si-CH_3$$
$$CH_3$$

Tetramethyl saline sulfonate (TMS)

$$CH_3$$
$$CH_3 - Si - CH_2 - CH_2 - CH_2 - SO_3Na$$
$$CH_3$$

Sodium, 3-(Trimethyl silyl) propane sulfonate: water soluble

NOTE: Maleic acid, Dimethyl sulfones, 1,4-BTM-d_4 and DSS-d_6 are other reference compounds used in Quantitative NMR

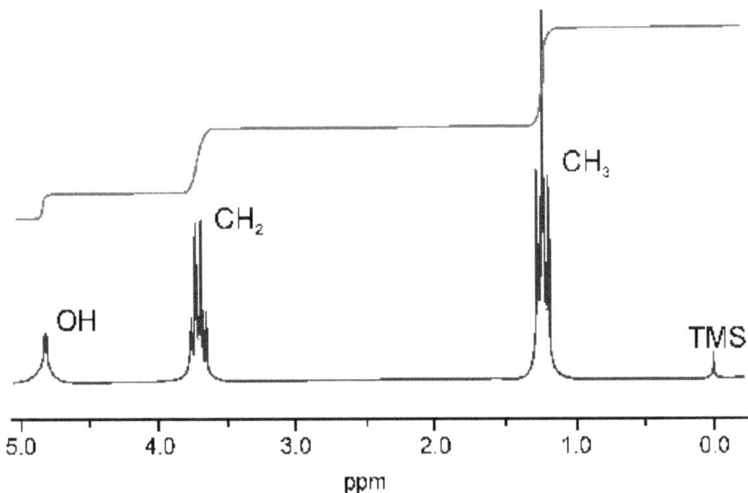

Figure 3.4 NMR spectrum of Ethanol.

Chemical Shifts

In NMR spectrum, X-axis is called chemical shift, and calculated from precessional frequency of sample proton in a sample molecule and reference (TMS) the following formula. The unit is parts per million. So different proton absorbs frequency at different energy, as they differ in precessional frequency at a given magnetic field (Bo).

$$\delta_{sample} = \left(\frac{v_{sample} - v_{reference}}{v_{reference}} \right) \times 10^6$$

Other formula are

- Chemical shift = Chemcal shift of Test proton - Chemcal shift of TMS
- Chemical shift in Tau value = 10 – delta value (ppm)
- Chemical shift (delta in ppm) = Shift of proton in HZ / Instrument frequency in MHZ

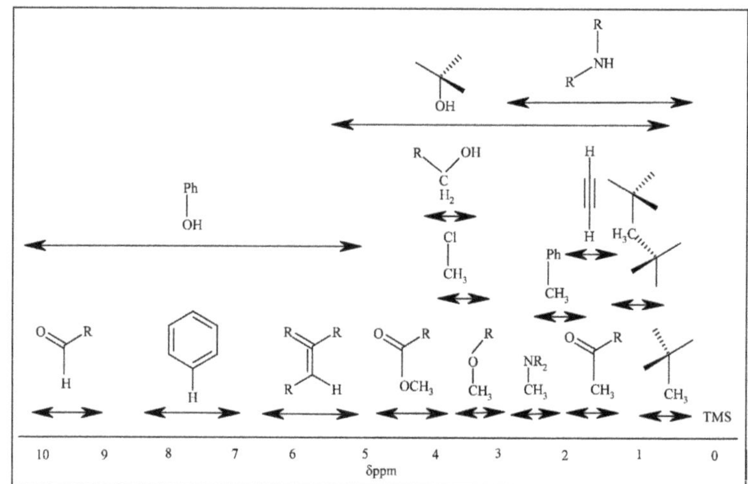

Figure 3.5A Chemical shifts of proton with respect to various functions.

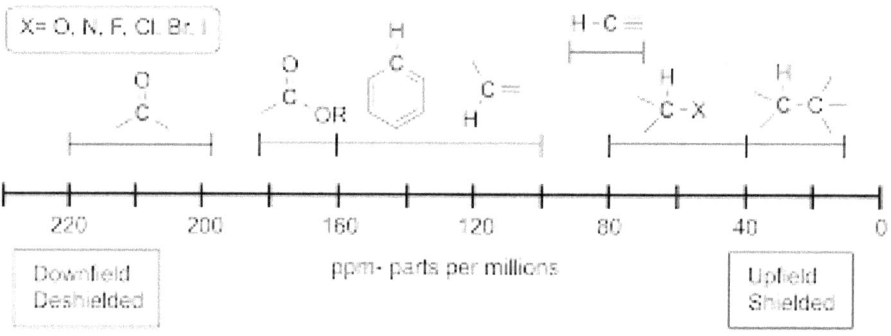

Figure 3.5B Chemical shifts of proton with respect to various functions (Up field is shielded and down field is deshielded.

- 0 ppm is the shielding zone or high field, where protons of SP3 hybridized carbon and electropositive zone
- Higher delta values are deshielding zone or low filed (low tau value = high delta value)
- The delta value (in ppm) increases (deshielding) with increase in proximity of proton to electronegative atoms like O, N, Pi bonds (Figure 3.5A and 3.5B) but exception for NH protons.
- Simple NMR spectra are recorded in solution (minimum 10%), and solvent protons must not be allowed to interfere.
- Deuterated (deuterium = ^{2}H, often symbolized as D) solvents especially for use in NMR are preferred, e.g. deuterated

chloroform, $CDCl_3$, and deuterated dimethyl sulfoxide, $(CD_3)_2SO$ (DMSO).

- However, a solvent without hydrogen, such as carbon tetrachloride, CCl_4 or carbon disulphide, CS_2, may also be used. But some time reactive.

NOTE:

Historically, deuterated solvents were supplied with a small amount (typically 0.1 %) of tetramethylsilane (TMS) as an internal standard for calibrating the chemical shifts of each analyte proton. But now deuterated solvents are now commonly supplied without TMS.

'Chemical shift values are not precise, but typical - they are to be therefore regarded mainly as orientational. Deviations are in ±0.2 ppm range, sometimes more. The exact value of chemical shift depends on molecular structure and the solvent in which the spectrum is being recorded. Hydrogen nuclei are sensitive to the hybridisation of the atom to which the proton is attached and to electronic effects. Nuclei tend to be deshielded by groups which withdraw electron density. Deshielded nuclei resonate at higher δ values, whereas shielded nuclei resonate at lower δ values'

*'Note that labile protons (-OH, -NH$_2$, SH) have no characteristic chemical shift. However such resonances can be identified by the disappearance of a peak when reacted with D$_2$O, as deuterium will replace a proton. This method is called a **D$_2$O shake**. Acidic protons may also be suppressed when a solvent containing acidic deuterium ions (e.g. methanol-d$_4$) is used'. Chemical shift values for Proton with respect to function is shown in table 3.1.*

Table 3.1 Chemical shift values for different protons

Functional Group	CH$_3$	CH$_2$	CH
CH$_2$R	0.8	1.3	1.6
C=C	1.6	2.0	2.6
C≡C	1.7	2.2	2.8
C$_6$H$_5$	2.3	2.6	2.9
F	4.3	4.4	4.8
Cl	3.0	3.4	4.0
Br	2.7	3.4	4.1
I	2.2	3.2	4.2

Table 3.1 contd...

Functional Group	CH$_3$	CH$_2$	CH
OH	3.3	3.5	3.8
OR	3.3	3.4	3.7
OC$_6$H$_5$	3.8	4.0	4.3
OCOR	3.6	4.1	5.0
OCOC$_6$H$_5$	3.9	4.2	5.1
OCOCF$_3$	4.0	4.4	/
CHO	2.2	2.4	2.5
COR	2.1	2.2	2.6
COOH	2.1	2.3	2.6
COOR	2.0	2.3	2.5
CONR$_2$	2.0	2.1	2.4
CN	2.1	2.5	3.0
NH$_2$	2.5	2.7	3.0
NR$_2$	2.2	2.4	2.8
NRC$_6$H$_5$	2.6	3.0	3.6
NR$_3^+$	3.0	3.1	3.6
NHCOR	2.9	3.3	3.7
NO$_2$	4.1	4.2	4.4
SR	2.1	2.5	3.1
SOR	2.6	3.1	--
=O (aliphatic aldehyde)	--	--	9.5
=O (aromatic aldehyde)	--	--	10

Interpretation

1. Check the NMR spectrum for the appearance signal for TMS at 0 ppm and don't consider the signal as a proton signal from the analyte.

2. Count the number of signal and examine for pattern

3. Sometime signal will appear without split (singlet) sometime split as two (doublet), three (triplet) etc. The spit intensity will be based on the following Pascal's triangle

4. The following is the Pascal triangle where n is number neighboring protons

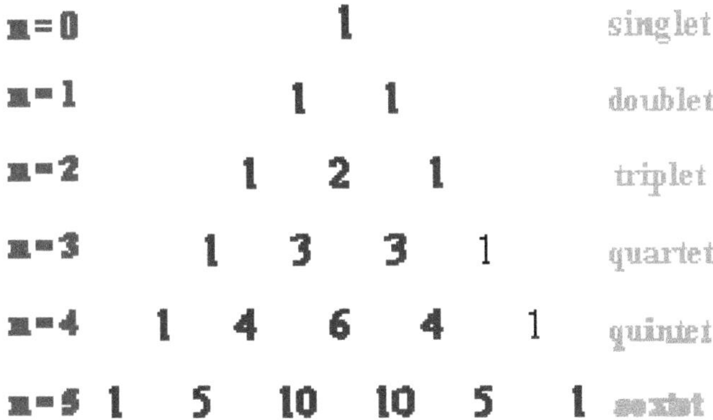

The split of signal is due coupling of proton with neighbor proton. The value between split is measured as Hz (coupling constant) which is important factor in assigning conformations and configuration.

N+1 Rule

Type of splitting is said to follow the "n+1 rule": a proton with n neighbors appears as a cluster of n+1 peaks.

Example 1: Ethanol

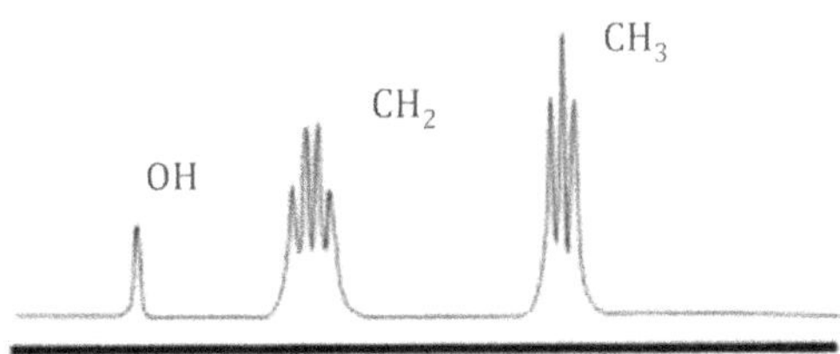

Figure 3.6 NMR spectrum of ethanol.

- Based on the chemical structure, there are three type of proton found, CH3, CH2, OH. So you can observe three signals (Figure 3.6).

- Among all OH proton appear to be high delta value indicated the deshielded of proton where as CH3 is more shielded as it appear near to TMS (low delta value).

- As per N+1 Rule, CH2 appeared as quartet and CH3 appeared triplet. But in case of OH still not split, owing to the paramagnetic property of the element. In general split for OH observed only for 100 % pure compounds and with very high NMR instrument frequency.

- Number of proton in each signal is estimated based on the intensity / AUC/ integral value (given by electronic integrator). Hence you can observe that the intensity order is CH3>CH2>OH.

Below is the example (Figure 3.7) for understanding the ratio of proton in NMR signals based on measurement.

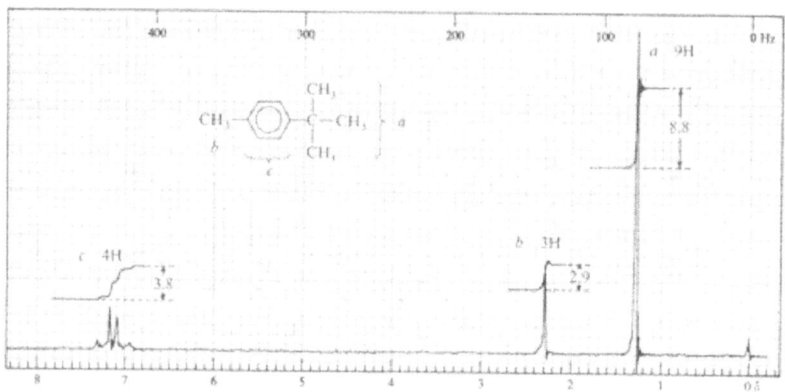

Figure 3.7 NMR spectrum of t-butyl toluene.

Example 2: 2-methylpropane, $(CH_3)_3CH$

$$H_3C-CH-CH_3$$
$$|$$
$$CH_3$$

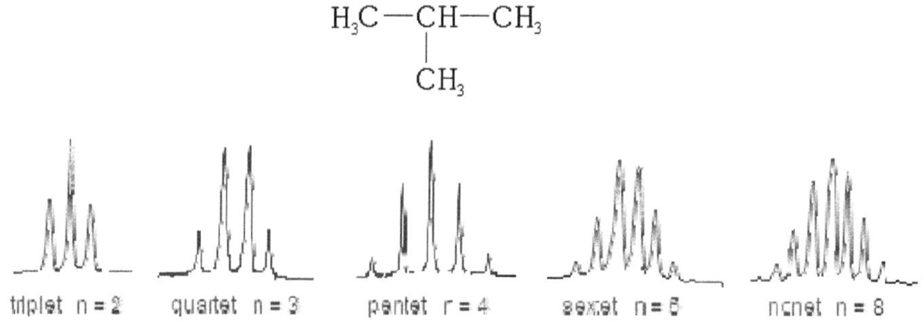

Figure 3.8 NMR spectrum of splitting of 2- methylpropane.

The CH proton is attached to three identical methyl groups (Figure 3.8). The C-H signal in the spectrum would be split into **ten** peaks according to the (n + 1) rule of multiplicity.

Note: 'The outer lines of the nonet (which are only 1/8 as high as those of the second peak) can barely be seen, giving a superficial resemblance to a septet. When a proton is coupled to two different protons, then the coupling constants are likely to be different, and instead of a triplet, a doublet of doublets will be seen. Similarly, if a proton is coupled to two other protons of one type, and a third of another type with a different coupling constant, then a triplet of doublets is seen. In the example below, the triplet coupling constant is larger than the doublet one. The analysis of such multiplets (which can get very much more complicated than the ones shown here) provides important clues to the structure of the molecule being studied'.

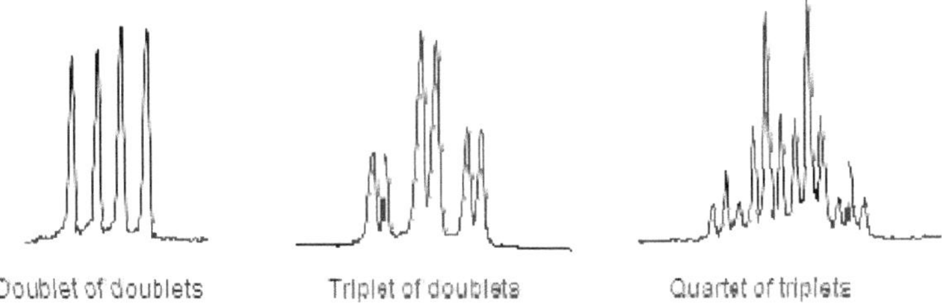

Figure 3.9 NMR spectrum of triplets and doubles.

Carbon Satellites and Spinning Sidebands

In few cases, small peaks may be shouldering the main H_1 NMR signals, and are not the result of proton-proton coupling, but due to the result from the coupling of H_1 atoms to an adjoining carbon 13 atom (Hetero-nuclear coupling). These small peaks are called as carbon satellites as they are small and appear around the main 1H peak i.e. satellite (around) to them. Carbon satellites are small because Carbon 13 only makes up about 1% of the atomic carbon content of carbon, the rest of the carbon atoms are predominantly NMR inactive Carbon 12.

if the main 1H-peak is a doublet then the carbon satellites will appear as miniature doublets, i.e. one doublet on either side of the main 1H-peak. Sometime other peaks can be seen around 1H peaks, these are known as spinning sidebands and are related to the rate of spin of an NMR tube. Carbon satellites and spinning sidebands should not be confused with impurity peaks

Example 1: NMR Spectrum of Ethanol (Figure 3.10)

- Integration height represents the number4 proton in one signal
- Each signal split in to triplet, quartet its depends on number of neighbor proton
- For example in Ethanol, CH3 Split three time, CH2 split four time based on N+1 Rule (where n is equal to number neighbor proton, In general OH involve in splitting only in high resolution and 100 % pure sample)
- 0 ppm is the signal of TMS.

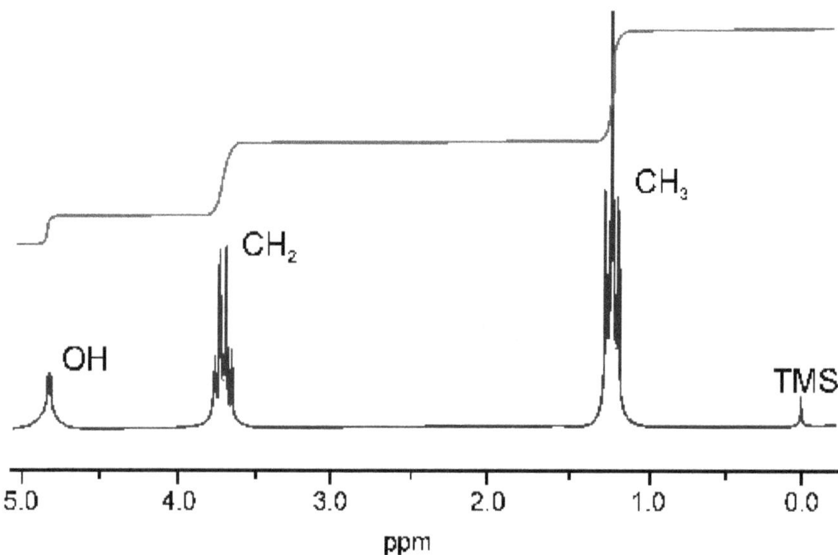

Figure 3.10 NMR spectrum of Ethanol.

Example 2:

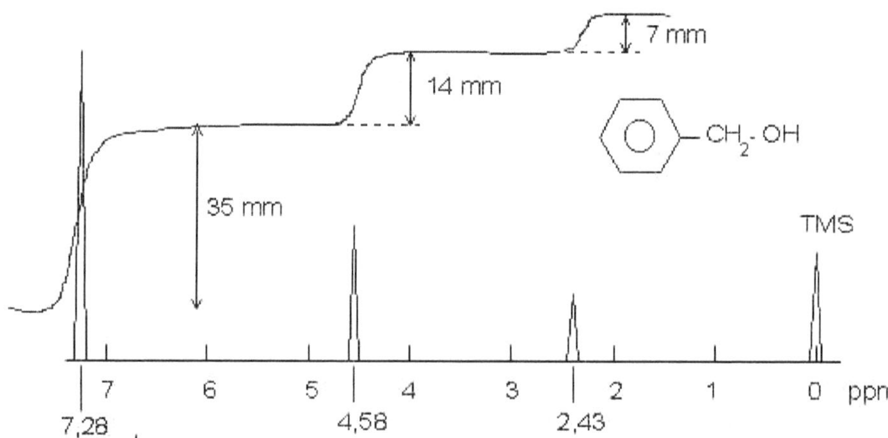

Figure 3.11 NMR spectrum of benzyl alcohol.

"Integer value of 35 mm is equal to 5 proton in benzene, so 14 mm is equal to 2 proton, and 7 mm is equal to one proton"

Example 3:

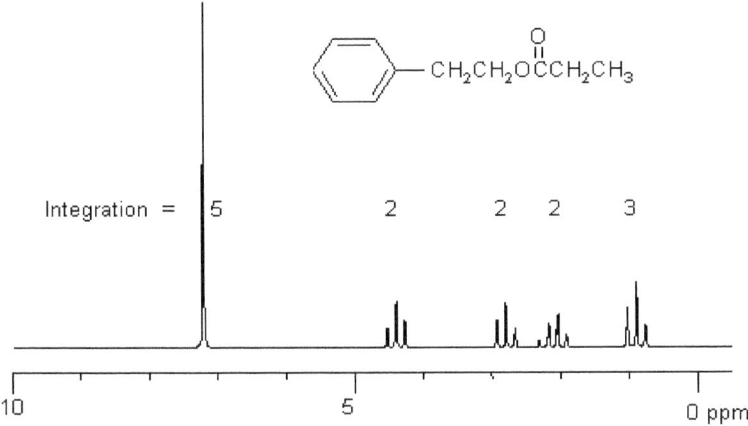

Figure 3.12 NMR spectrum of Phenethyl acetate.

If the solvent is free from TMS, no signal for TMS is observed.

Example 4:

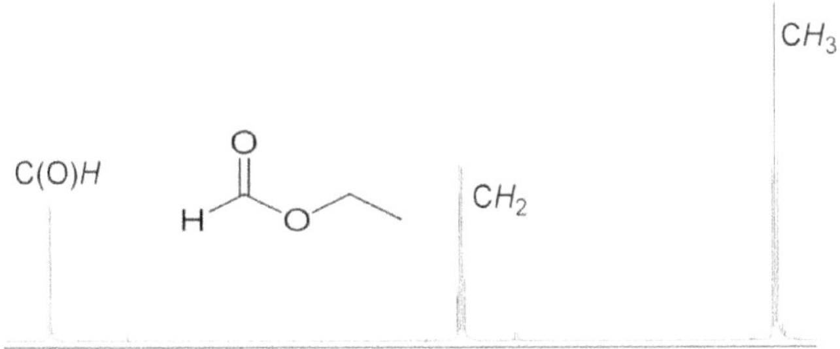

Figure 3.13 NMR spectrum of propanoic acid.

Example 5:

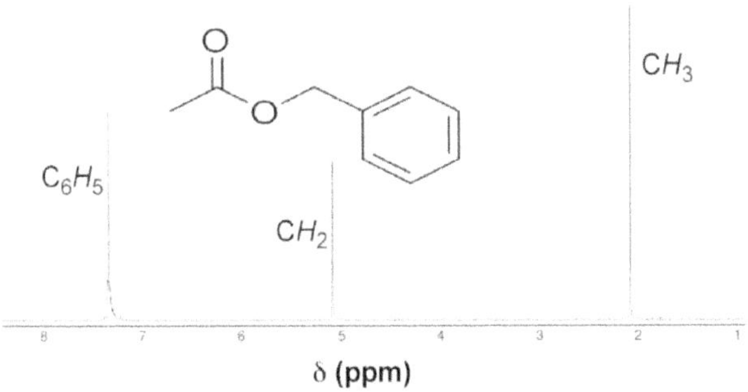

Figure 3.14 NMR spectrum of benzyl acetate.

Authentication of Paracetamol by H^1-NMR

In the structure, there four major types of protons (NH, CH3, Aromatic, OH) out all CH3 is shielded appeared near to TMS (low delta value). DMSO-d6 is the residual solvent proton. Aromatic proton has multiplicity (complex) due to dissimilar Para substitution (Figure 3.15).

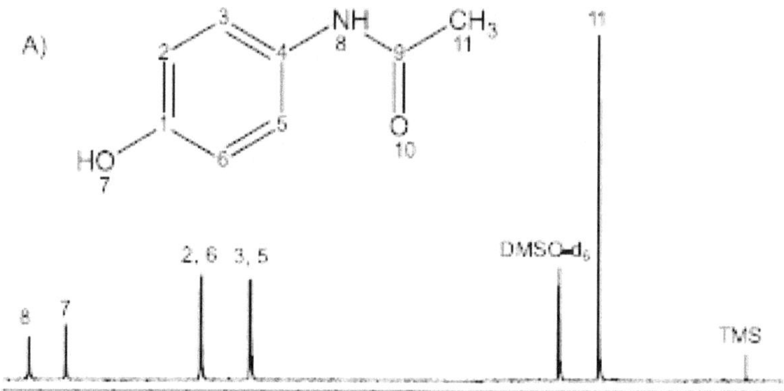

Figure 3.15 NMR spectrum of paracetamol.

Example of Nitro Phenol: You can observe that aromatic system appeared as complex (delta value 7-8 ppm due to non- symmetric substitution. 9.8 ppm is due to highly deshielded OH proton (Figure 3.16).

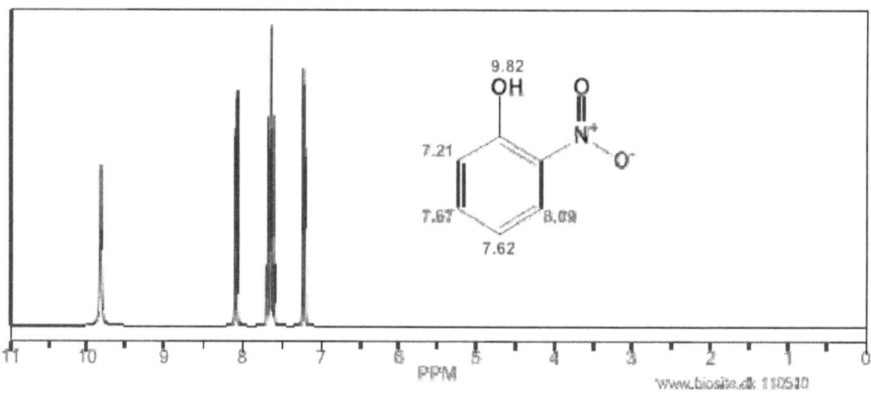

Figure 3.16 NMR spectrum of nitro phenol.

Detection of Impurities by Proton NMR

In the following Proton NMR spectrum (Figure 3.17) of 4-methyl acetophenone there are two signals (coupled) at 2-3 ppm are due to two methyl protons. 7-8 ppm is for phenyl proton. A small signal at 3.5 ppm indicate the impurity (preferably a aliphatic proton).

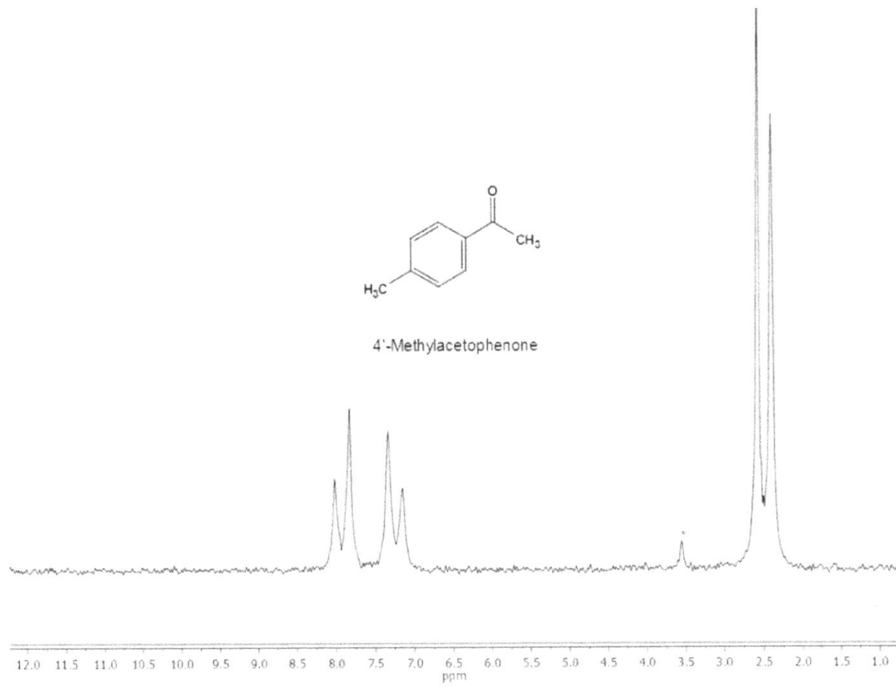

Figure 3.17 NMR spectrum of 4-methyl acetophenone.

Identification NH Proton and Conformational Structures

In the given below Proton NMR spectrum (Figure 3.18) of Aminorex you can find the broad signal (c) for NH2 group it is due to the quadruple interaction. The doublet-doublet (dd) is due to d' and e' proton coupling among b, d, e proton. In the same way b complex signal is due to coupling effect with a, d, e.

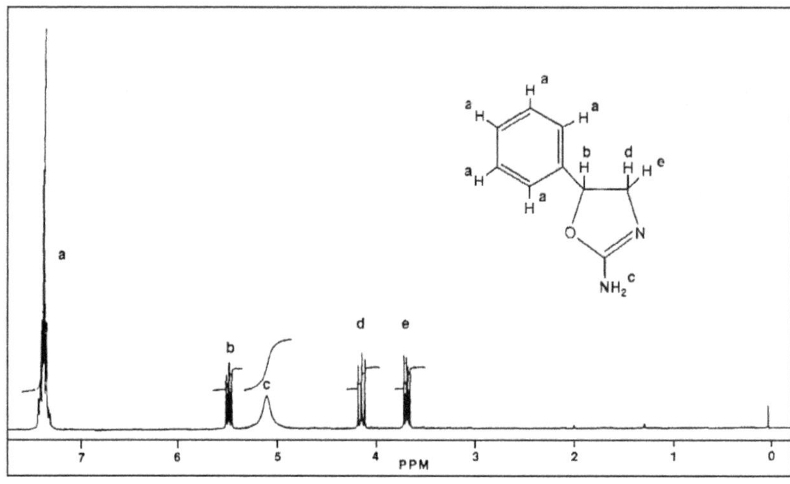

Figure 3.18 NMR spectrum of aminorex.

Determination of ratio of two product by H¹- NMR (applicable to estimation of impurity also)

The integral of each ^{1}H-NMR signal is relative to the number of equivalent ^{1}H-atoms in the sample that generate that signal. This information can be used to calculate the ratio of two or more molecules in the same spectrum, assuming that the at least one signal for each molecule is adequately resolved. In the following spectrum (Figure 3.19) ratio vinyl proton (for Product A) and methylene proton (for product B) can be considered for calculation of ratio.

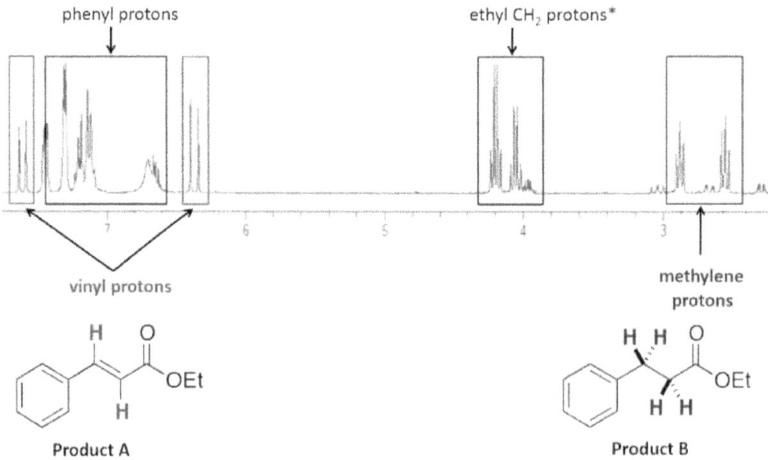

Figure 3.19 NMR spectra of vinyl protons (Product A) and methylene protons (Product B).

Isomer assignment by H^1-NMR

It is done by the coupling constant (J – value). J-Value is defined as the Hz value measure between two adjacent split, due to coupling. In the below figure consider that two type of protons (Ha and Hb), where Ha appears as triplet and Hb appears as quartet. Then coupling constant is measured as Hz indicated as 'X' in the figure. The X value vary from proton to proton like cis, trans, vinyl, ortho, meta, para, etc (Figure 3.20).

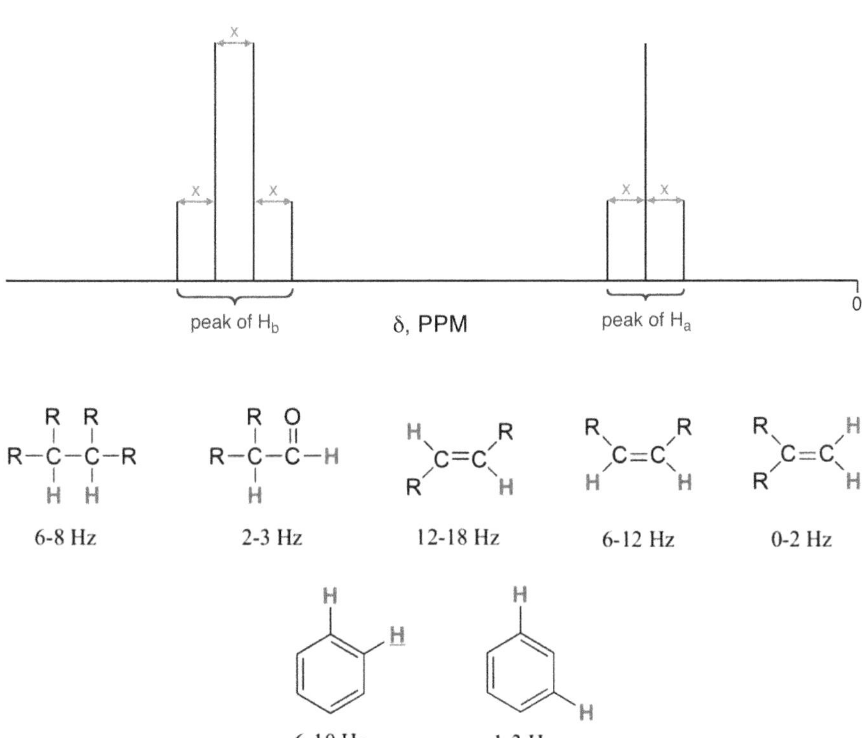

Figure 3.20 J – values or coupling constants in **H^{1}NMR** spectra of isomers.

CIS Trans - Isomers by H¹- NMR

Example: Cis-stilbene appears at up field than trans stilbene

Trans isomer
more downfield

Cis isomer more upfield

<------------------->

<---------------->

---

ppm

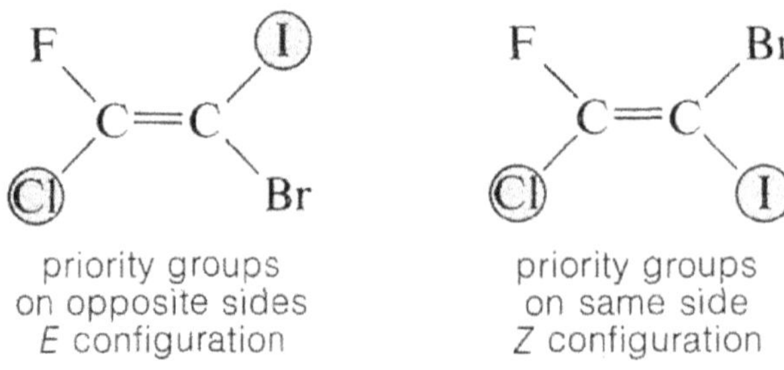

cis, δ = 6·49

trans, δ = 6·99

Coupling constant (J- Value) is the indicator for Cis and Trans: Based on the value it has to be assessed. J value for CIS is less when compare to Trans.

$^3J_{HH}$ = 9 Hz

Cis–

$^3J_{HH}$ = 14 Hz

Trans–

E-Z Configuration

It is a kind of geometrical isomerism (E - is similar to TRANS and Z is similar to CIS).

priority groups
on opposite sides
E configuration

priority groups
on same side
Z configuration

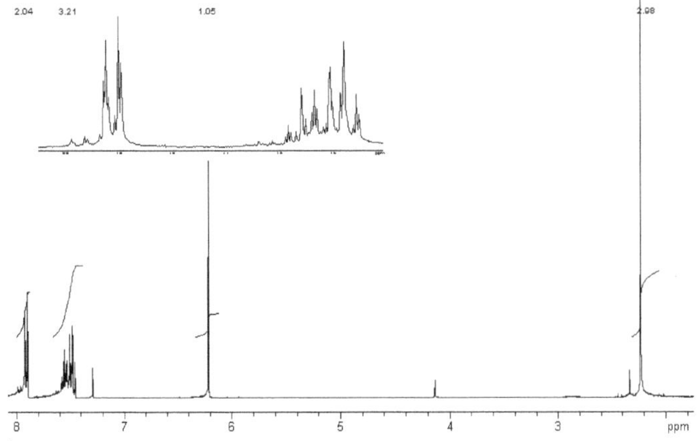

Optical Isomerism by H1-NMR

NMR spectroscopy can be used assign absolute configuration of stereoisomers such as *cis* or *trans* alkenes, *R* or enantiomers, and *R, R* or *R,S* diastereomers. The NMR spectrum of enantiomers mixture can help to quantify the each enantiomer by means of optical purity. It can be assessed by integrating the area under the NMR peak corresponding to each stereoisomer. NOTE: Accuracy of integration usually improved by chiral derivatizing agent with a nucleus other than hydrogen or carbon and then reading the heteronuclear NMR spectrum: for example fluorine-19 NMR or phosphorus-31 NMR. Mosher's acid contains a -CF_3 group, so if the adduct has no other fluorine atoms, the ^{19}F NMR of a racemic mixture shows just two peaks, one for each stereoisomer.

Excercise 1 ($C_6H_5COCH_2COCH_3$)

Figure 3.21 NMR spectrum of 1-phenyl-1,3-butanedione.

Exercise 2 $(CH_3)_2CHCH_2OH$

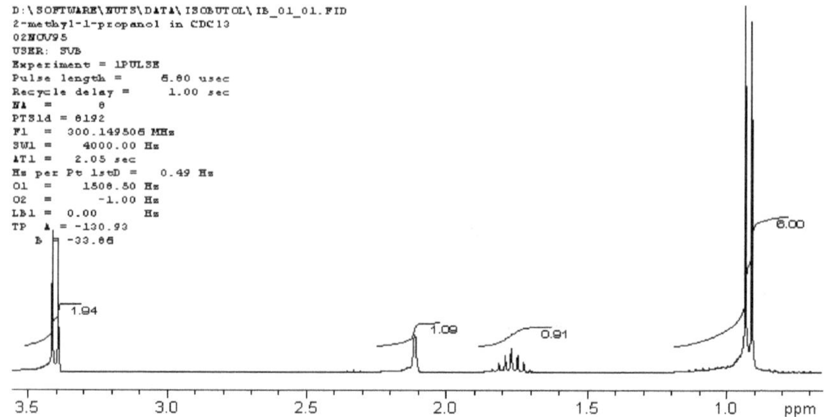

Figure 3.22 NMR spectrum of 2-methyl 1-propanolol.

Exercise 3 $CH_3C_6H_4CHO$

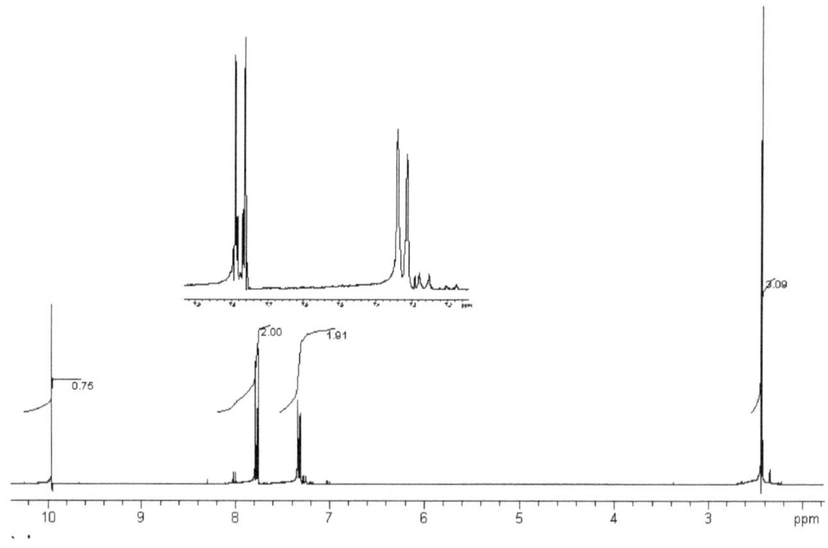

Figure 3.23 NMR spectrum of 2-methylbenzaldehyde.

C^{13} - NMR Interpretation

- The NMR spectrum of C^{13} always with noise and is a decoupled spectrum

- No splitting pattern is considered. All signals appears as non-spilt lines

- Height of the C^{13} signal is directly proportional to number hydrogen atom attached to the carbon, it is due to nuclear over Hauser effect.

- Thus signal for C=O will be very less when compare to CH3.

- Number of line signals is equal to the number carbon atom in structure.

- In case of symmetry molecule the spectrum simple and single signal appears for magnetically equivalent carbon.

Example: C^{13}-NMR spectrum of Acetone (Figure 3.24A)

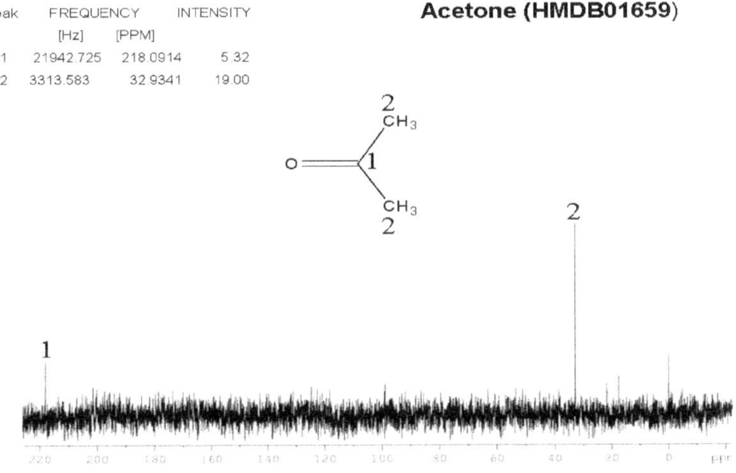

Figure 3.24A C^{13}-NMR spectrum of acetone.

In Figure 3.24A, Signal 2 is for 2 carbons (2CH3). The intensity is very high due to the more number of hydrogen (Nuclear Hauser effect (NOE)). Signal 1 is for C=O, sometime C=O signal may be mixed with Noise (intensity of Noise and intensity of C=O will be same). The chemical shift values are shown in Figure 3.24B.

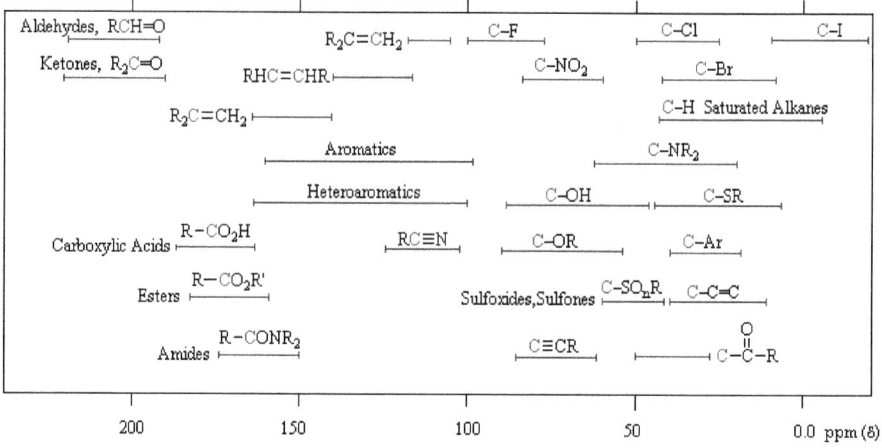

Figure 3.24B Chemical shift values for various carbons (C¹³) in NMR Spectrum.

Example 1:

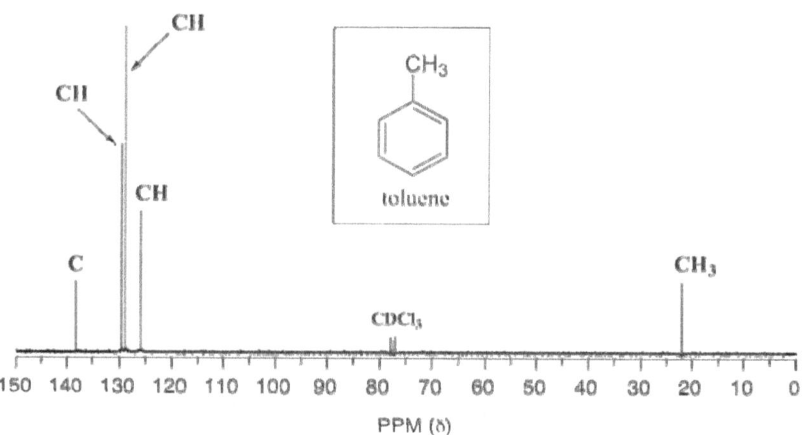

Figure 3.25 C¹³-NMR spectrum of toluene.

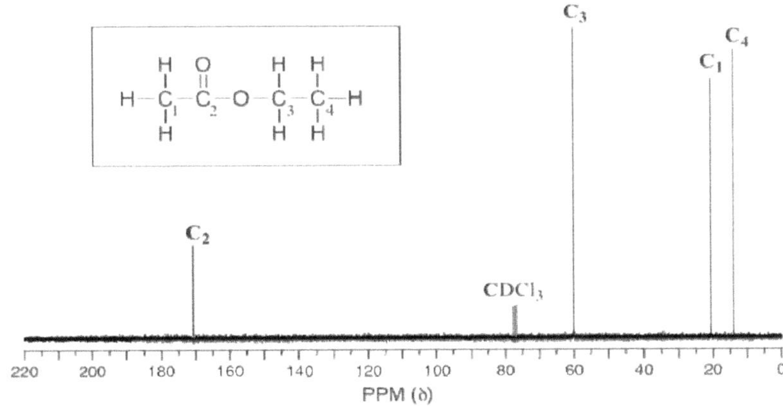

Figure 3.26 C^{13}-NMR spectrum of ethyl acetate (Example).

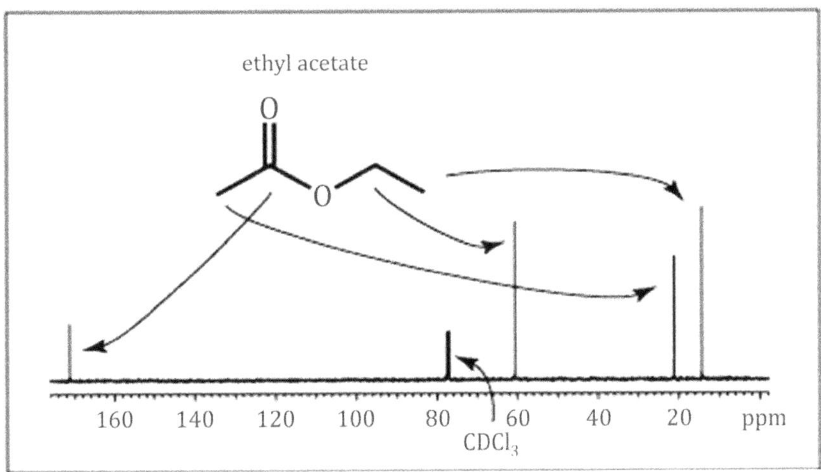

Figure 3.27 C^{13}-NMR spectrum of Ethyl acetate (Example).

Exercise Section: Interpret the following C^{13}- NMR spectra,

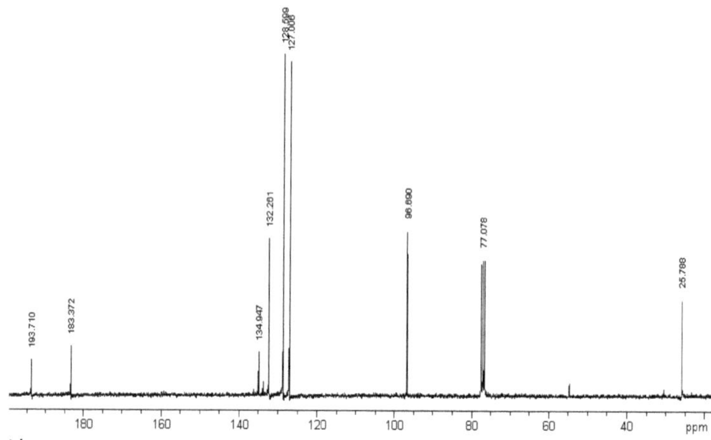

Figure 3.28 NMR spectrum of Benzoyl acetone.

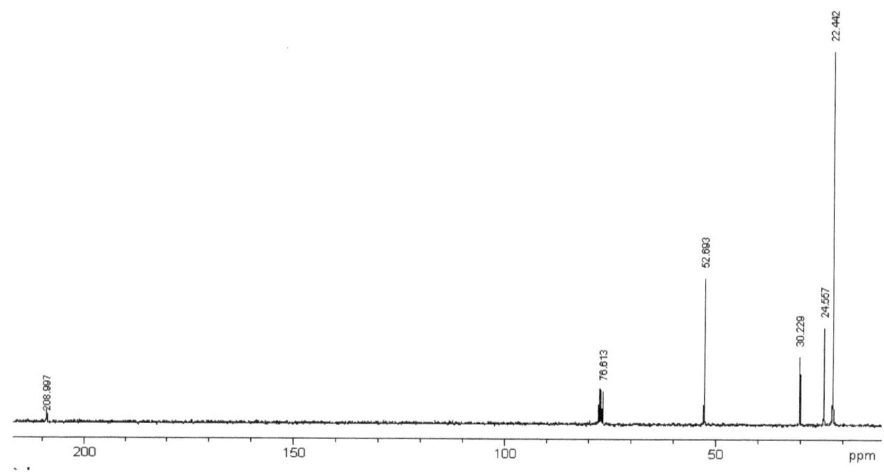

Figure 3.29 NMR spectrum of 4-methyl – 3- pentanone.

2D- NMR Spectrum

The construction of a 2D experiment involves an indirect evolution time t_1 and a mixing sequence along with normal spectrum (1D NMR). This scheme has shown below (Figure 3.30).

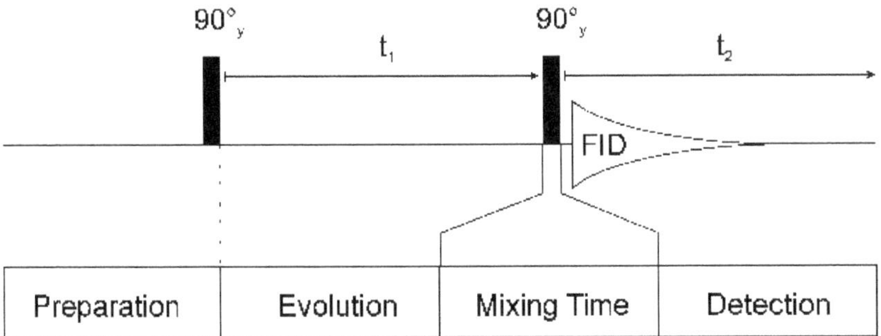

Figure 3.30 2D – NMR Experiment.

- The nulcei preparation,

- Free evolution with t1: During this time the magnetization is labeled with the chemical shift of the first nucleus to a second one.

- **Mixing time:** Mixing sequences depends on the mechanisms for magnetization transfer so called scalar coupling or dipolar interaction (NOE), in which data are acquired at the end of the experiment (detection, often called direct evolution time). During this time the magnetization is labelled with the chemical shift of the second nucleus.

- **Detection the result:** acquisition time (t2) will be converted to frequency spectrum using FID (free induction decay).

- Two dimensional FT yields the 2D spectrum with two frequency axes. If the spectrum is homonuclear (both axis signals of the same isotope (usually ¹H). it has a characteristic topology because the spectrum is detected at different evolution time using two frequencies. The sample 2D spectrum is shown below. In which A, B are two signal responsible (diagonal peak) for two type of proton in the structure (diagonal position). X indicates the interaction of both A and B. X (cross peak) is the indicator for the interaction of proton and environment. 2D spectrum is a diagonal symmetry spectrum (Figure 3.31).

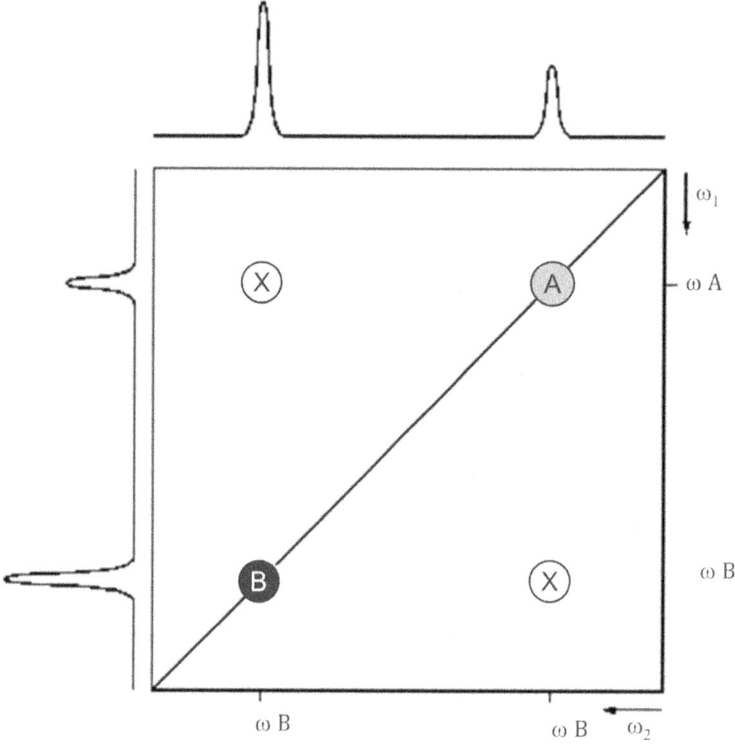

Figure 3.31 2D- NMR Spectroscopy.

Example of 2 D NMR spectrum H¹-H¹ COSY: the following spectrum (Figure 3.32) shows the 2D – proton NMR spectrum for Phenyl ring proton (2H, 3H, 4H, 5H). (COSY: Correlation spectroscopy)

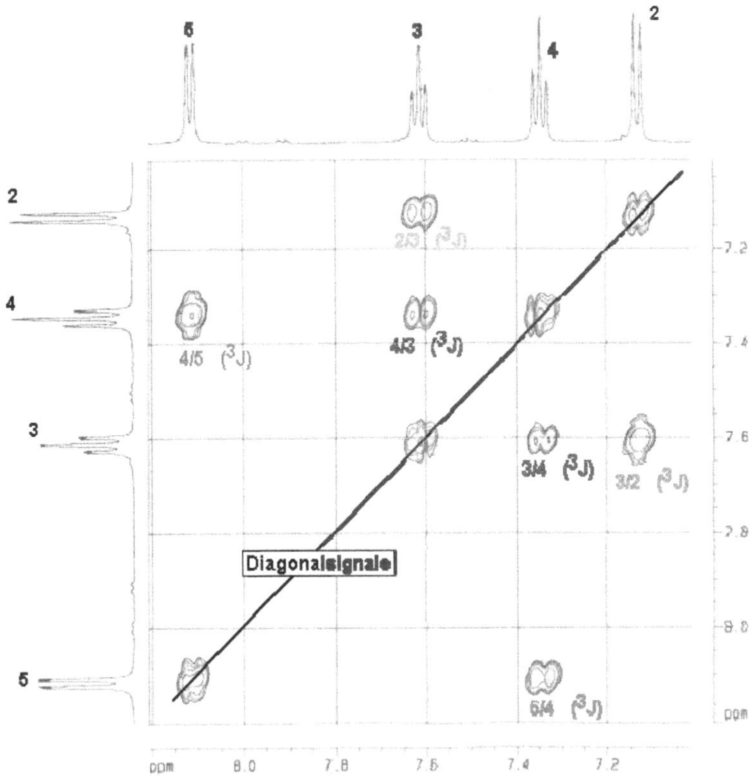

Figure 3.32 Homonuclear 2D NMR spectrum H¹-H¹ COSY.

- Diagonal signal indicate the interaction of same proton during mixing.
- Signals appeared above and below are due to other interaction of neighbor nuclei effect.
- The proton of signal 4 has interaction with proton signal 5.
- The proton of signal 4 has interaction with proton signal 3.
- The proton of signal 2 has interaction with proton signal 3.
- NOTE: proton 2 and 5 are away so, no interaction was found.

2D NMR - H¹-C¹³ COSY

The following spectrum (Figure 3.33) shows the heteronuclear 2D spectrum of H1-C13 Correlation spectrum. In which X axis is the proton spectrum while Y axis is C13 spectrum. Interpolation of X axis signal to Y axis signal will indicate the interaction effect and 3D position assignment of atom.

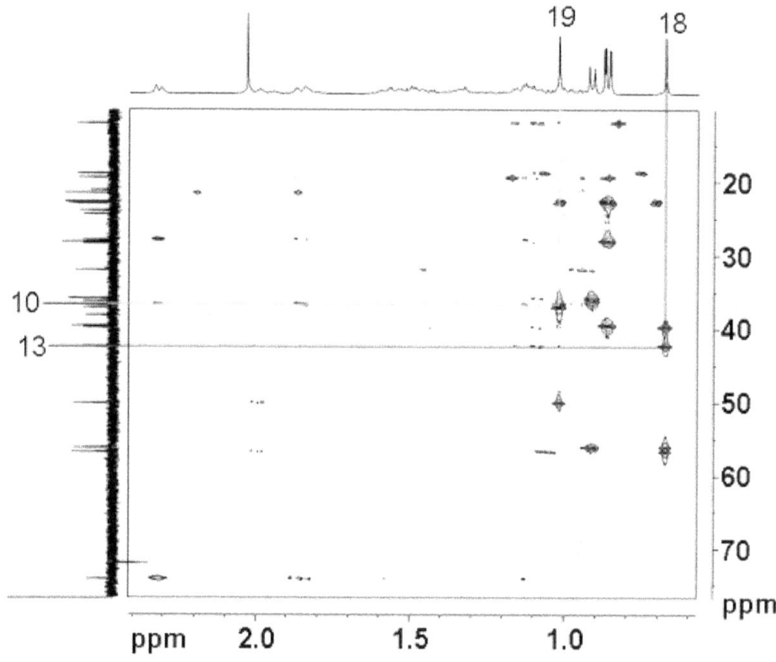

Figure 3.33 Heteronuclear 2D spectrum of H^1-C^{13} COSY.

The **Heteronuclear Single Quantum Coherence** (HSQC) or **Heteronuclear Single Quantum Correlation** (HETCOR) experiments are used frequently in NMR spectroscopy of organic molecules and are of particular significance in the field of proton NMR. The experiment was first described by Geoffrey Bodenhausen and D. J. Ruben in 1980. The resulting spectrum is two-dimensional with one axis for ^1H and the other for a *heteronucleus* (an atomic nucleus other than a proton), most often ^{13}C or ^{15}N. The spectrum contains a peak for each unique proton attached to the heteronucleus being considered.

- The HSQC experiment is a highly sensitive 2D-NMR experiment and was first described in a ^1H–^{15}N system, but is also applicable to other nuclei such as ^1H–^{13}C system.

- The basic scheme of this experiment involves the transfer of magnetization on the proton to the second nucleus, which may be ^{15}N or ^{13}C, via an INEPT (Insensitive nuclei enhanced by polarization transfer) step.

- After a time delay (t_1), the magnetization is transferred back to the proton via a retro-INEPT step and the signal is then recorded.

- In HSQC, a series of experiments is recorded where the time delay t_1 is incremented. The ^{1}H signal is detected in the directly measured dimension in each experiment, while the chemical shift of ^{15}N or ^{13}C is recorded in the indirect dimension which is formed from the series of experiments.

- The following spectrum is a HSQC NMR spectrum for protein (Figure 3.34), in which N^{15}in Y axis and H^1 nuclei is at X-axis.

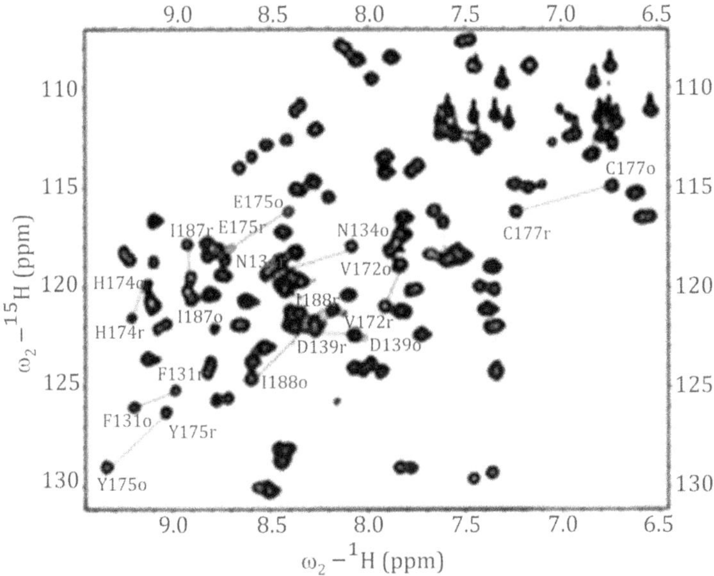

Figure 3.34 Heteronuclear single-quantum correlation spectroscopy.

Chapter 4

Electron Spin Resonance Spectroscopy

It is similar to that of proton NMR, but here microwaves are used to change the spin state of electron from ground state (-1/2) to excited state (+1/2) under the magnetic field (Bo) (Figure 4.1).

Only odd electron containing compounds (radicals, transition elements) responds to absorption process of Microwave (9.5 to 10.5 GHz) under 0.35 tesla of magnetic strength. Microwaves are produced by klystron oscillator.

The internal standard used is DPPH. **DPPH** is a common abbreviation for an organic chemical compound 2,2-diphenyl-1-picrylhydrazyl. It is a dark-colored crystalline powder composed of stable free-radical molecules. DPPH has two major applications, both in laboratory research: one is a monitor of chemical reactions involving radicals, most notably it is a common antioxidant assay, and another is a standard of the position and intensity of electron paramagnetic resonance signals.

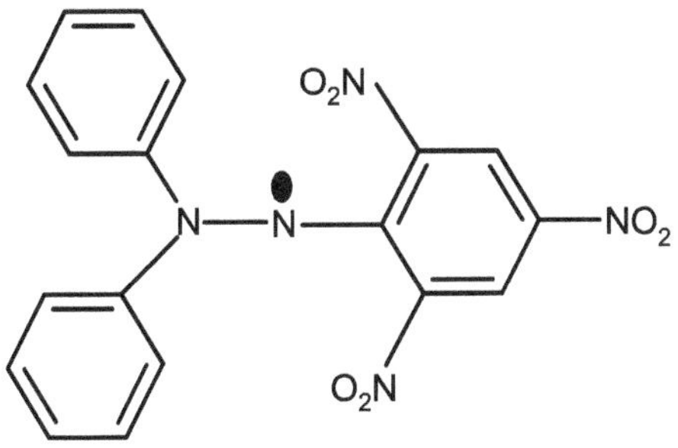

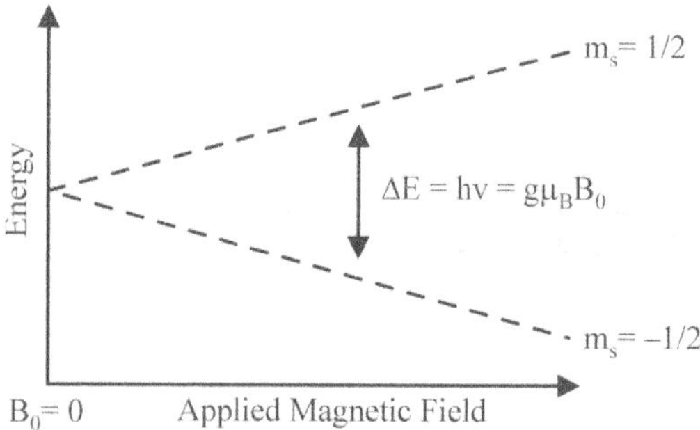

Figure 4.1 Electron spin change in ESR Spectroscopy.

The electron's magnetic moment aligns itself either parallel (ms = −1/2) or antiparallel (ms = +1/2) to the field, each alignment having a specific energy due to the Zeeman effect

$$E = m_s g_e \mu_B Bo$$

Where,

- 'g' is the electron's so-called g-factor (2.003 is the value for free electron)
- μB is the Bohr magneton.

Instrumentation: The following Figure 4.2 shows schematic diagram of ESR instrumentation.

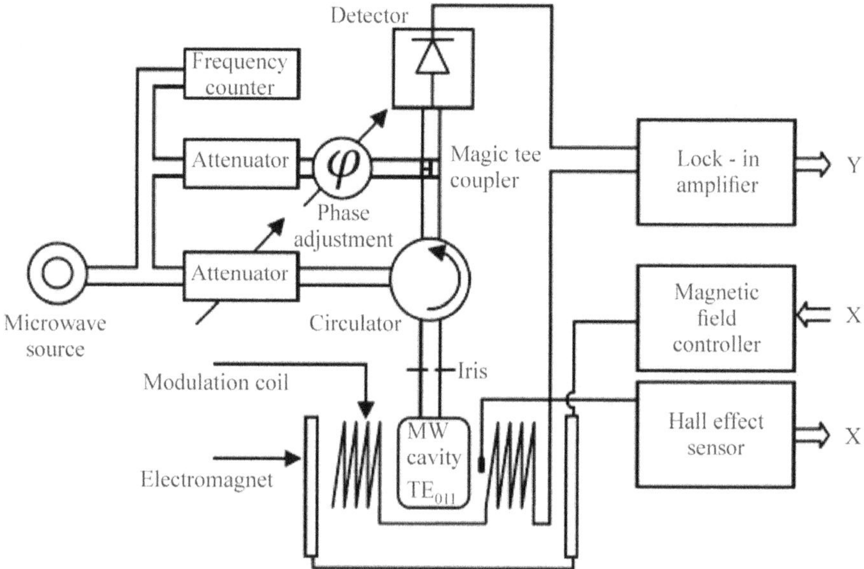

Figure 4.2 ESR instrumentation.

ESR Absorption spectrum: It is similar to that of UV spectrum, where X axis is magnetic scan and Y axis is absorbance of microwave (Figure 4.3). Same like splitting is observed for ESR signal, it is similar to that of proton NMR (N+1 Rule). This is called as hyperfine coupling (due to the neighbour nuclei)

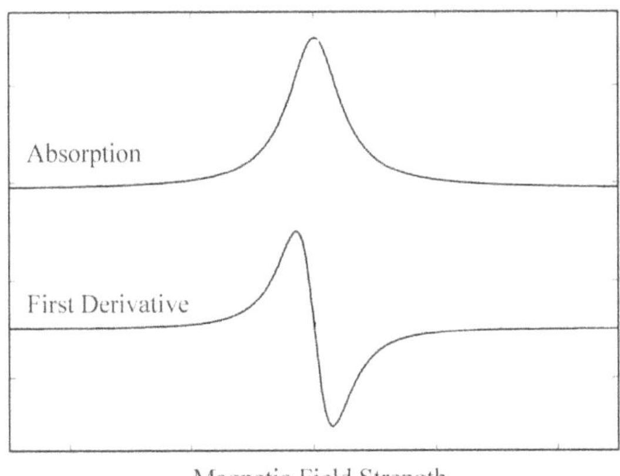

Figure 4.3 ESR Absorption spectrum.

Example 1: ESR signal for CH_3 radical (appears as four split (N+1 rule) because of 3H)

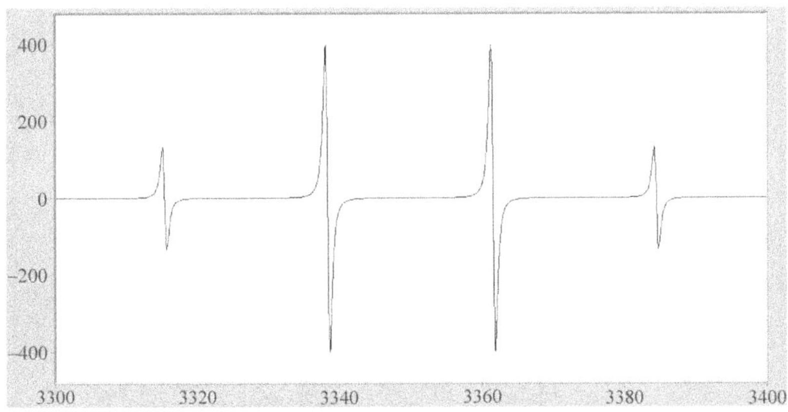

Figure 4.4 ESR signal for CH_3 radical.

NOTE: spectrum at the right shows that the three ^1H nuclei of the CH_3 radical give rise to 2MI + 1 = 2(3)(1/2) + 1 = 4 lines with a 1:3:3:1 ratio.

Example 2: Consider the methoxymethyl radical, $H_2C(OCH_3)$. The two equivalent methyl hydrogens will give an overall 1:2:1 EPR pattern, each component of which is further split by the three methoxy hydrogen's into a 1:3:3:1 pattern to give a total of 3×4 = 12 lines, a triplet of quartets.

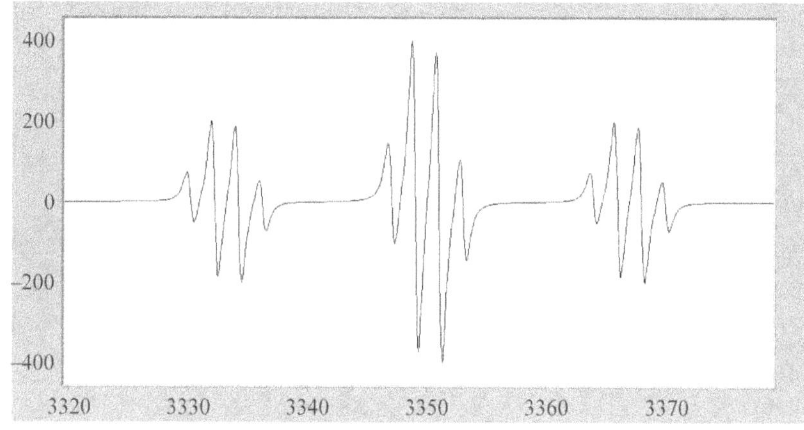

Figure 4.5 ESR signal for Methoxymethyl radical.

Examine the following?

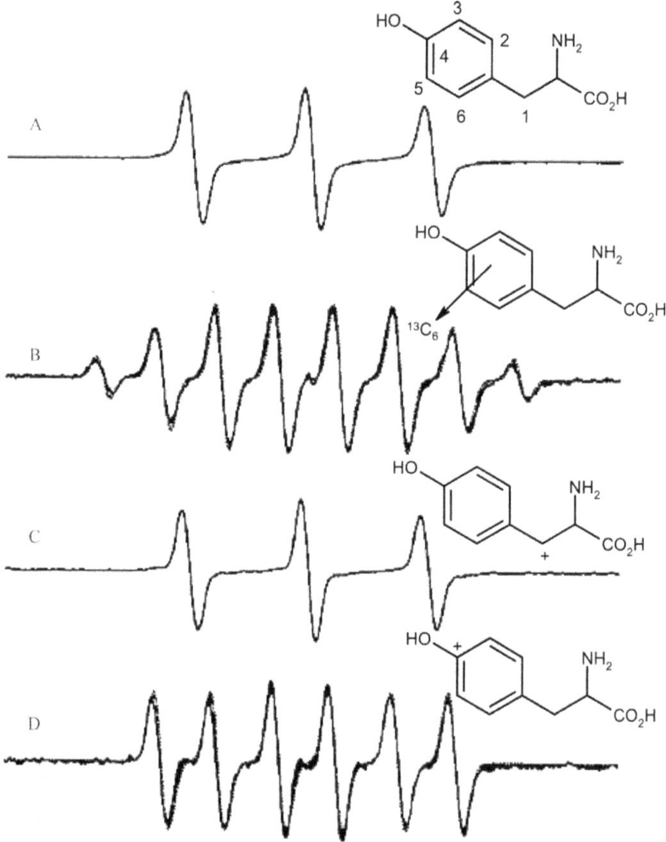

Figure 4.6 Example of ESR spectra.

Chapter 5

Mass Spectroscopy and Interpretation

Mass spectrometry is a most important analytical technique used to

- find out the molecular weight,
- identify unknown compounds within a sample,
- Isotope ratio
- Elucidate the structure and
- Study of different isomers

Now days the mass spectrum is coupled with Liquid chromatography as exist as LC-MS or LC-MS/MS or LC-(MS) n. This hyphenated technique is currently a most suitable for identification and quantification of drug, metabolites and other biomolecules in biological fluid. LC-MS/MS (tandem spectroscopy) serve as a tool in Clinical trials for estimating various pharmacokinetic parameters and drug interaction studies.

Principle

The mass spectrometry involves the conversion of the sample molecule into gaseous ions, with or without fragmentation, which are then characterized by their mass to charge ratios (m/z) and relative abundances. The conversion of neutral gas molecule to positively charged molecule is ionization process (Figure 5.1), it is attained by different ionization techniques

- Electron impact (EI) – 70 eV used to ionize
- Chemical ionization (CI)- Reagent gas (methane, ammonia etc)
- Fast atom bombardment ionization (FAB) – For soft molecule based on the collision between high velocity Xe or Ar gaseous molecule.
- Electro-spray Ionization (ESI)– Based on voltage at spray nozzles used for polar molecule in LC-MS
- Atomic pressure chemical ionization (APCI)- for Non –polar molecule in LC-MS

- Matrix assisted Laser desorption ionization (MALDI)- based on the sample-matrix (sample mixed with urea, nicotinic acid etc.) which was ionized by the irradiation of LASER.

- M+1 (quasi molecular ions) ions are more common in all techniques except Electron impact ionization.

- A simple mass spectrometer is shown in Figure 5.2.

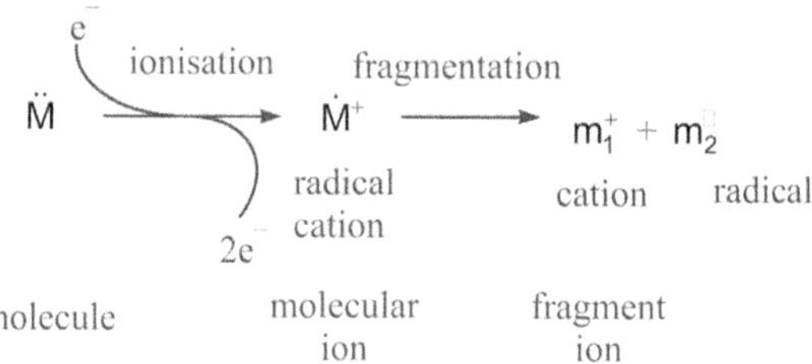

Figure 5.1 Fragmentation in Mass spectrometry.

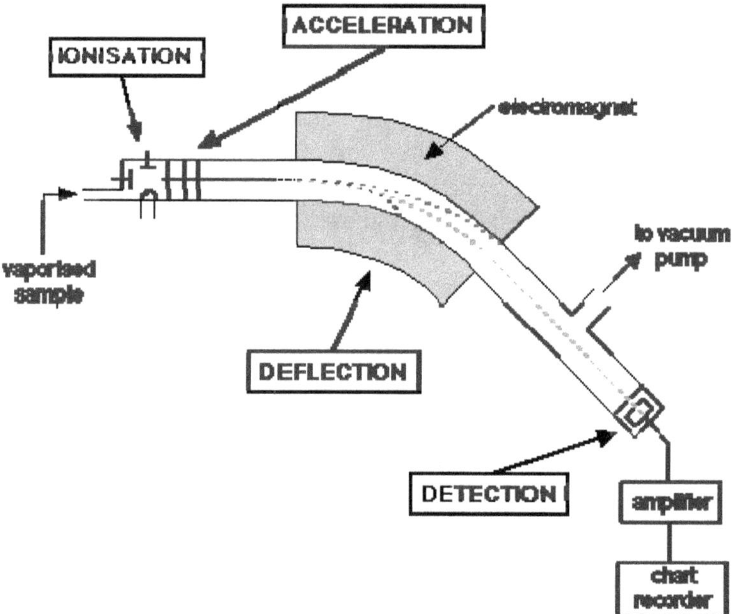

Figure 5.2 Instrumentation of Mass spectrometer.

The choice of ionization technique is based on the sample nature with respect to molecular weight,

- polarity,
- thermo/electro labile nature of molecule,
- the intensity of molecular ion (parent ion) and
- product ion (fragment ion).

There different type of mass spectrometers depends on our requirement.

- LC-MS (single quadrupole)
- LC-MS/MS (triple quadrupoles)
- LC-Q (ion traps, linear ion traps)
- LC-Q-TRAPS (quadrupole linear ion traps)
- LC-TOF-MS (time-of-flight)
- MALDI-TOF-MS
- Q-TOF-MS (quadrupole time-of-flight)
- FT-MS (Fourier Transform)

As a result of formed ions mixture will be separated by analyzer of mass spectrum. (Most common example of analyzers, are quadrupole analyzer, Time of flight analyzer (TOF).

Based on the fact that different ions will possess different translational energy, as a result ions will move in different radius (under field), different oscillations (in quadrupole analyzer) and different velocity (Time of flight). Accordingly the abundance of ions (% in Y axis) will be scanned by m/z (mass per charge ratio).

Mass Spectrum

The following spectrum (Figure 5.3) is an original spectrum of mass spectrum (usually with lots of base line noise).

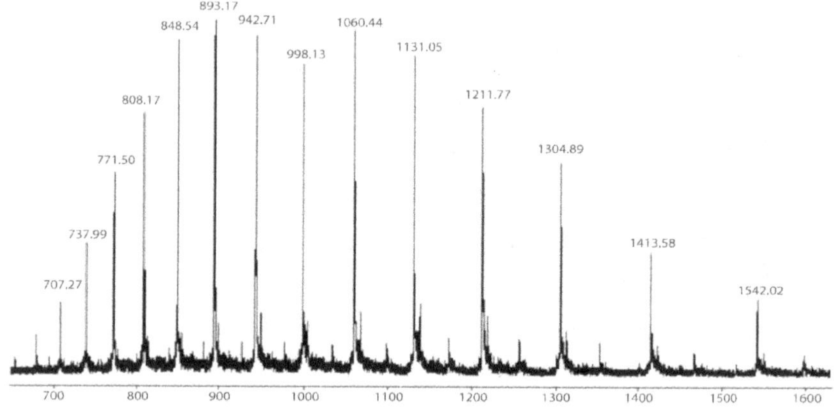

Figure 5.3 Mass spectrum.

Bar Graph of Mass Spectrum (Noise are removed)

While conversion of mass spectrum of bar graph representation of mass spectrum (compare with Figure 5.3), the intensity of less than 0.5 % abundance are removed (Figure 5.4).

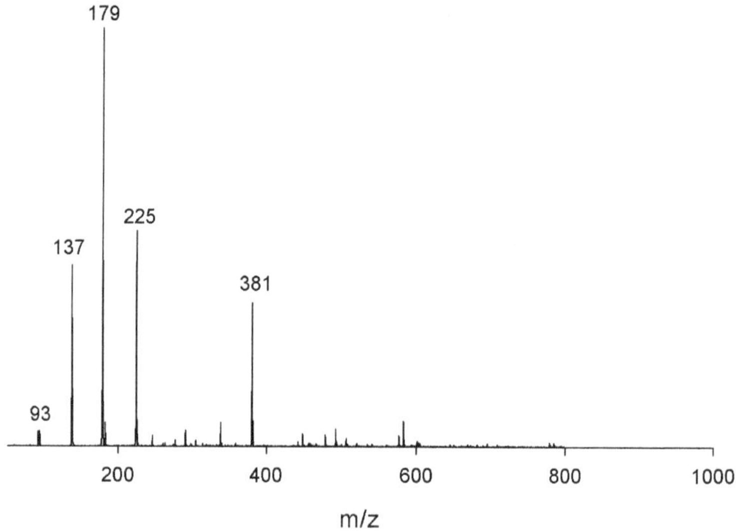

Figure 5.4 Bar Graph of Mass spectrum.

A typical LC-MS/MS Spectrum (Figure 5.5)

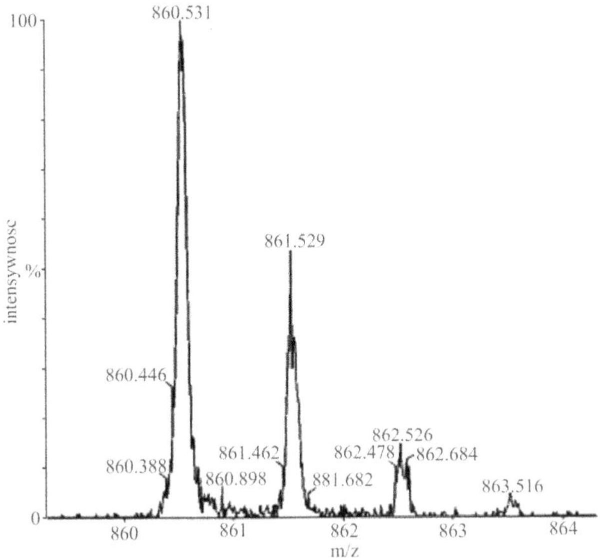

Figure 5.5 LC-MS/MS spectrum.

Different Peaks in Mass Spectrum

1. Molecular ion (parent peak – highest m/z)
2. Base peak (100 %)
3. Fragment peaks (lower m/e value than molecular ion peak
4. Isotope peak (M+1, M+2) – should not be confused with quasi-molecular ion peak.
5. Metastable ion peak (m/z value with decimal value.. example 36.4, its due to abnormal translation al energy of ions which has ionized at analyzer instead at ionization chamber). If M* is metastable peak, the following formula will be used for calculation

$$M^* = M_2{}^2/M_1$$

e.g. $C_5H_9{}^+$ (m/z = 69) $\rightarrow$ $C_3H_5{}^+$ (41) + C_2H_4 (28)

Calculated $m^* = (41)^2/69 = 24.36$, observed $m^* = 24.4$

Example 1:

- In the following figure 5.6, m/z 58 is parent ion, indicated the molecular weight of the compound is 58.
- m/z 59 indicate the M+1 isotope peak due to C13 or H2 isotopes.
- m/z 43 is the most stable ions appeared as base peak (100 %)

- No metastable ions formed during fragmentation.

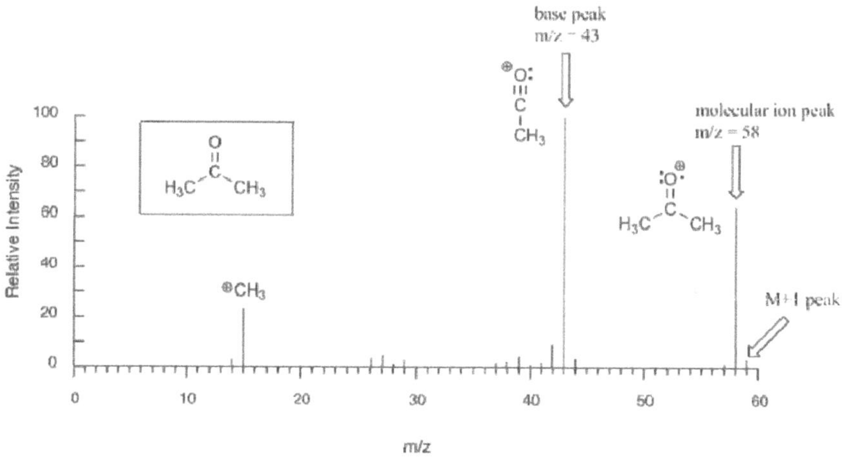

Figure 5.6 Mass spectrum of Acetone.

Example 2:

- In the following figure 5.7 m/z 106 is parent ion, indicated the molecular weight of the compound is 106.

- m/z107 indicate the M+1 isotope peak due to C13 or H2 isotopes.

- m/z 91 is the most stable ions appeared as base peak (100 %)

- No metastable ions formed during fragmentation.

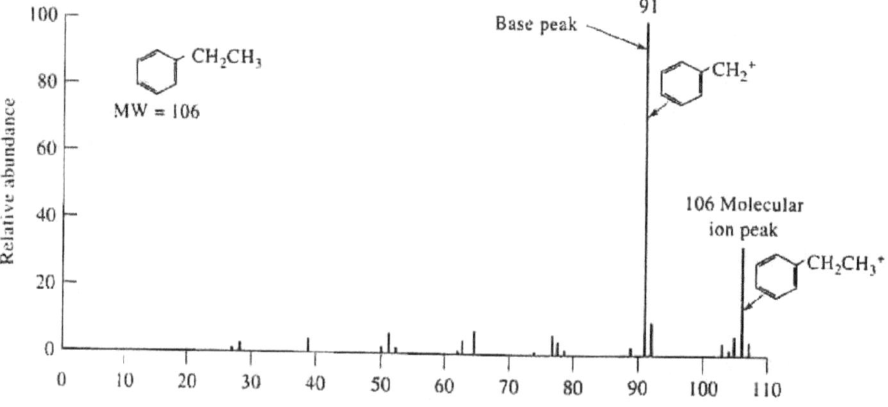

Figure 5.7 Mass spectrum of Ethyl benzene.

Identify the various peaks in the below spectrum (figure 5.8)?

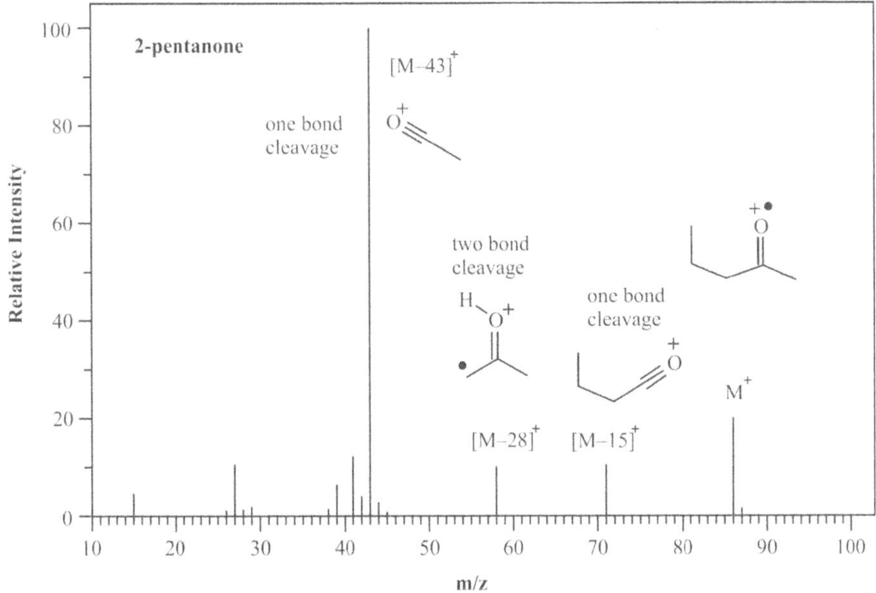

Figure 5.8 Mass spectrum of 2-pentanone.

% Abundance of Isotope Peak

Its depend up on % abundance of a particular atom. For example chlorine and bromine. **Chlorine:** 75.77% ^{35}Cl and 24.23% ^{37}**Cl** and **Bromine:** 50.50% ^{79}Br and 49.50%. In Figure 5.9, the % ratio of peak intensity for bromine at m/z 79 and m/z 81 determine the isotope abundance. In the same way for Chlorine in Figure 5.10.

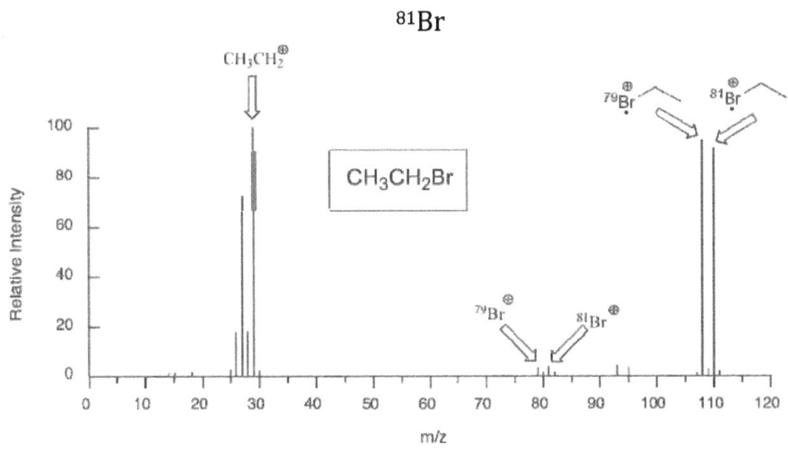

Figure 5.9 Mass spectrum of Ethyl bromide.

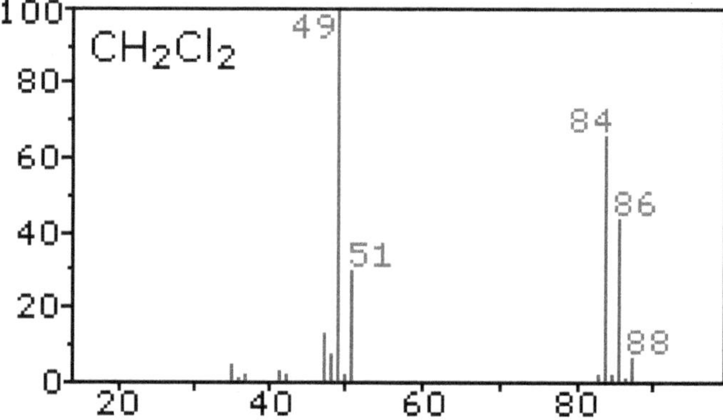

Figure 5.10 Mass spectrum of Dichloromethane.

Adduct Products: the following spectrum (Figure 5.11) shows the presence of Adducts of molecular ion m/e 212 (appeared as quasi m molecular ion (m/e 213) with sodium (m/e 235) and potassium (m/e 251). It's very common in LC-MS due to mobile phase.

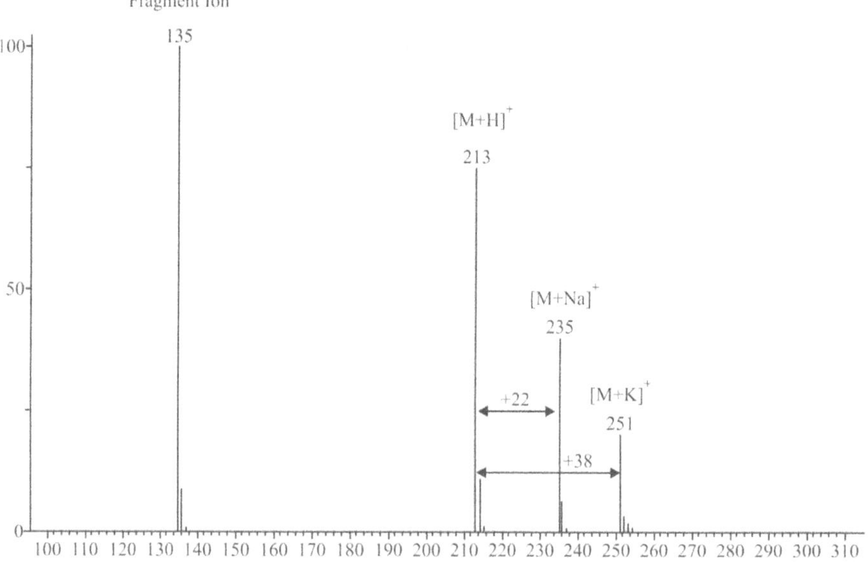

Figure 5.11 LC-MS of Adduct products.

Alcohol

- An alcohol's molecular ion is small or non-existent.
- Cleavage of the C-C bond next to the oxygen usually occurs.
- A loss of H_2O may occur.

Example: 3-Pentanol ($C_5H_{12}O$) with MW = 88.15 (the following spectrum shows (Figure 5.12) the fragment ions only. Because the spectrum was not scanned for parent ions)

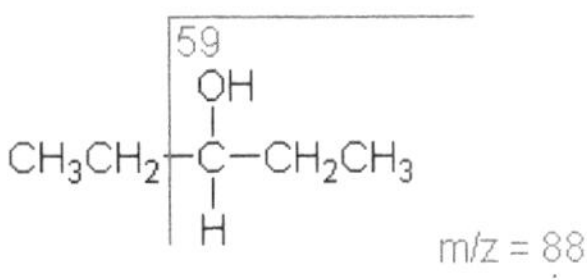

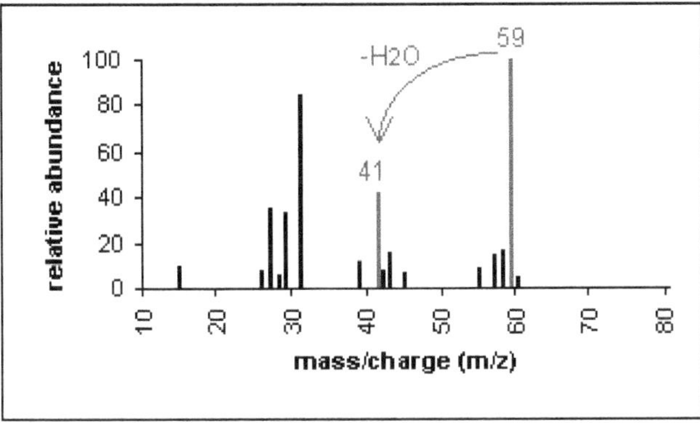

Figure 5.12 Mass spectrum of 3-Pentanol.

Aldehyde

- Cleavage of bonds next to the carboxyl group results in the loss of hydrogen (molecular ion less 1)
- The loss of CHO (molecular ion less 29).
- Example: 3-Phenyl-2-propenal (C_9H_8O) with MW = 132.16 (Figure 5.13)

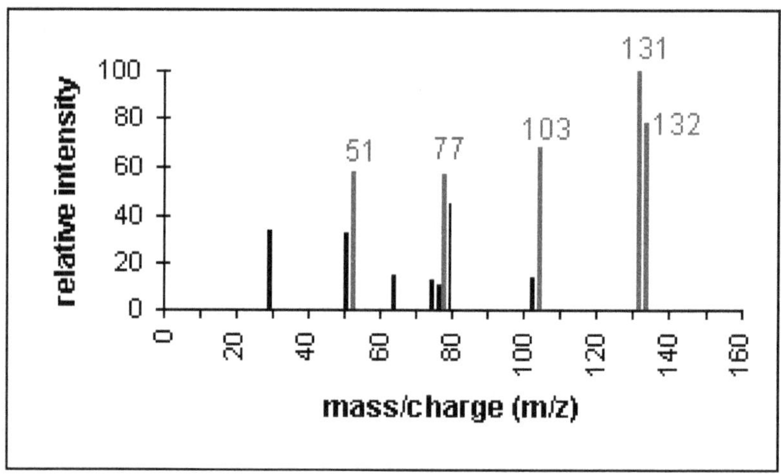

Figure 5.13 Mass spectrum of 3-Phenyl-2-propenal.

Alkane

- Molecular ion peaks are present, possibly with low intensity.
- The fragmentation pattern contains clusters of peaks 14 mass units apart (which represent loss of (CH2)nCH3).
- Hexane (C6H14) with MW = 86.18 (Figure 5.14)

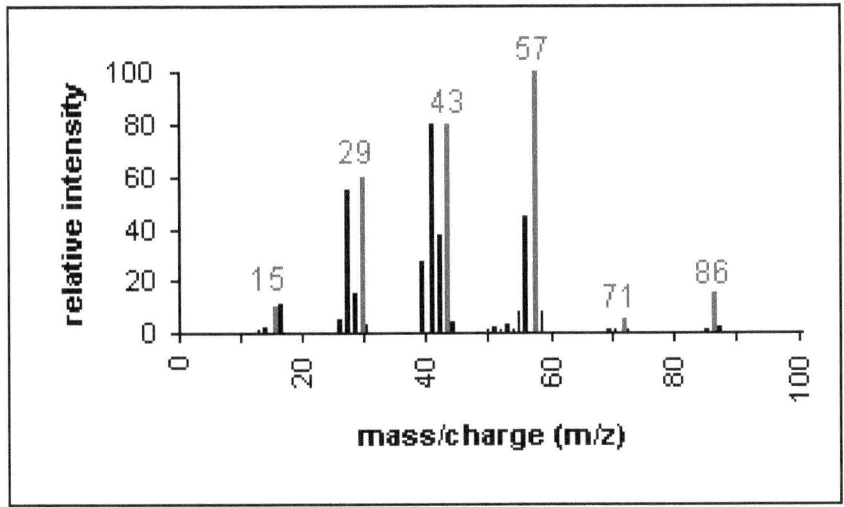

Figure 5.14 Mass spectrum of n-hexane.

Amide

- Primary amides show a base peak due to the McLafferty rearrangement.
- 3-Methylbutyramide ($C_5H_{11}NO$) with MW = 101.15 (Figure 5.15)

Amine

- Molecular ion peak is an odd number.
- Alpha-cleavage dominates aliphatic amines.
- n-Butylamine (C4H11N) with MW = 73.13 (Figure 5.16)

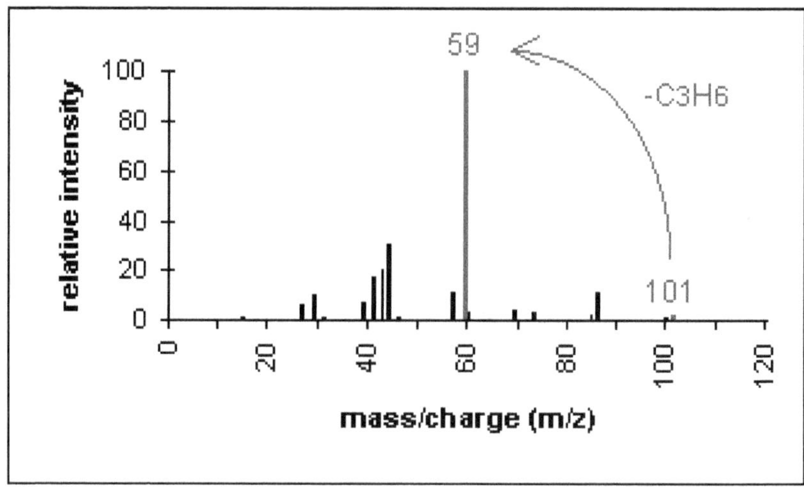

Figure 5.15 Mass spectrum of 3-Methylbutyramide.

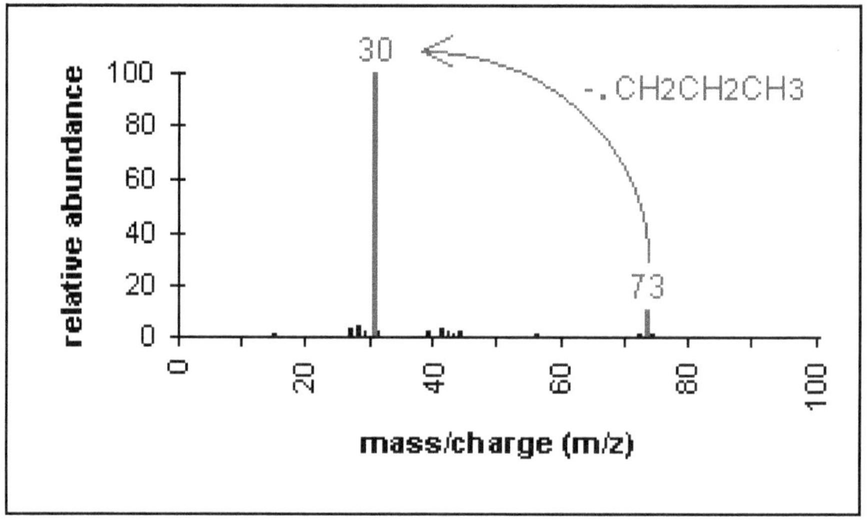

Figure 5.16 Mass spectrum of n-Butylamine.

- Another example is a secondary amine shown below.
- Again, the molecular ion peak is an odd number.
- The base peak is from the C-C cleavage adjacent to the C-N bond.
- n-Methylbenzylamine ($C_8H_{11}N$) with MW = 121.18 (Figure 5.17)

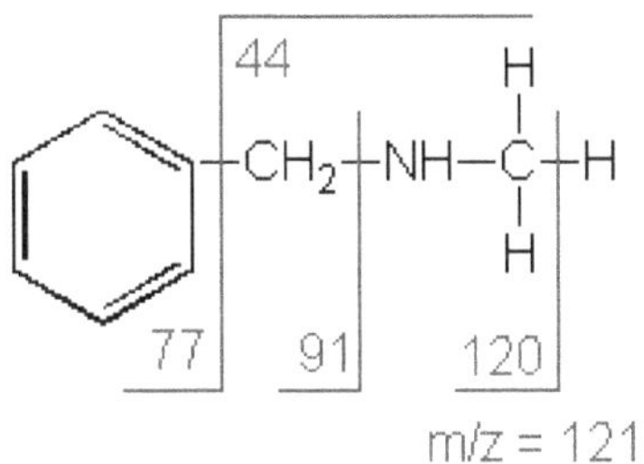

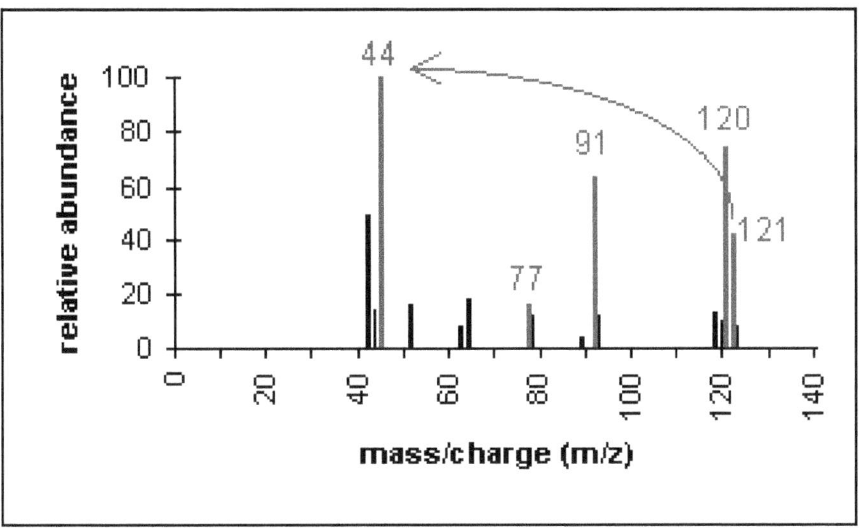

Figure 5.17 Mass spectrum of n-Methylbenzylamine.

Aromatic

- Molecular ion peaks are strong due to the stable structure.
- Naphthalene ($C_{10}H_8$) with MW = 128.17 (Figure 5.18)

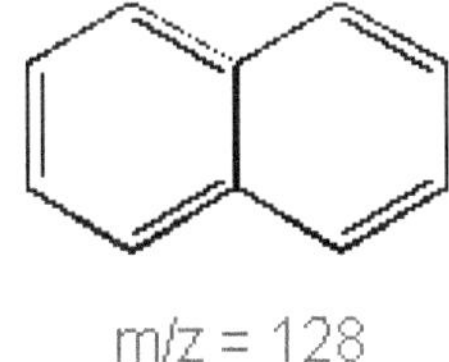

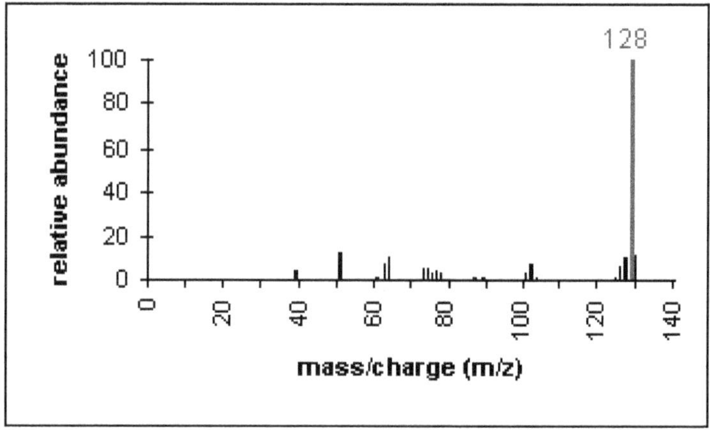

Figure 5.18 Mass spectrum of Naphthalene.

Carboxylic Acid

- In short chain acids, peaks due to the loss of OH (molecular ion less 17).

- COOH (molecular ion less 45) are prominent due to cleavage of bonds next to C=O.

- 2-Butenoic acid ($C_4H_6O_2$) with MW = 86.09 (Figure 5.19)

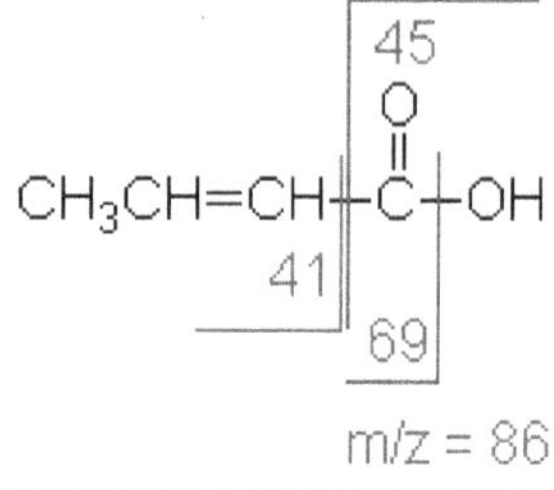

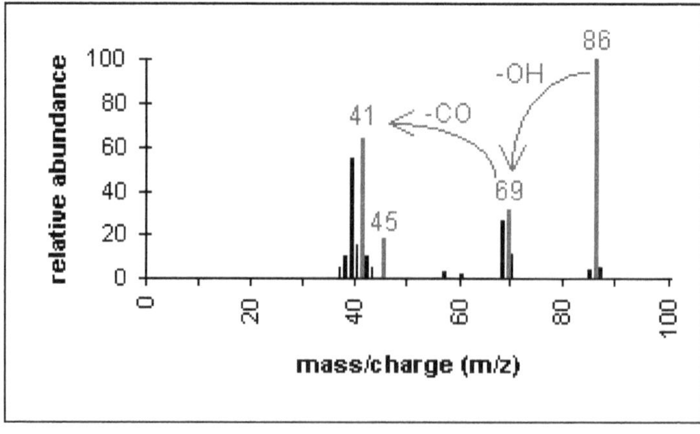

Figure 5.19 Mass spectrum of 2-Butenoic acid.

Ester

- Fragments appear due to bond cleavage next to C=O (alkoxy group loss, -OR) and hydrogen rearrangements.
- Ethyl acetate ($C_4H_8O_2$) with MW = 88.11 (Figure 5.20)

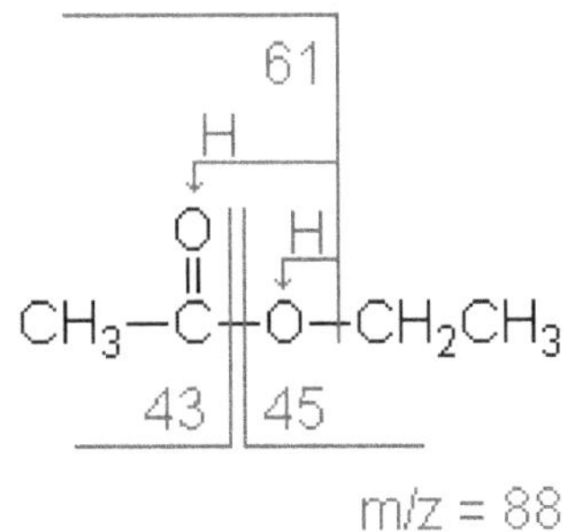

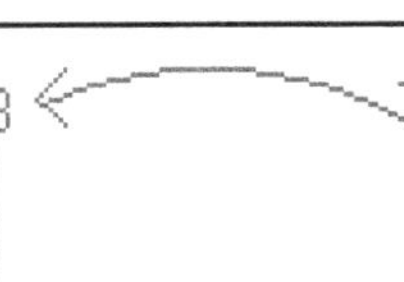

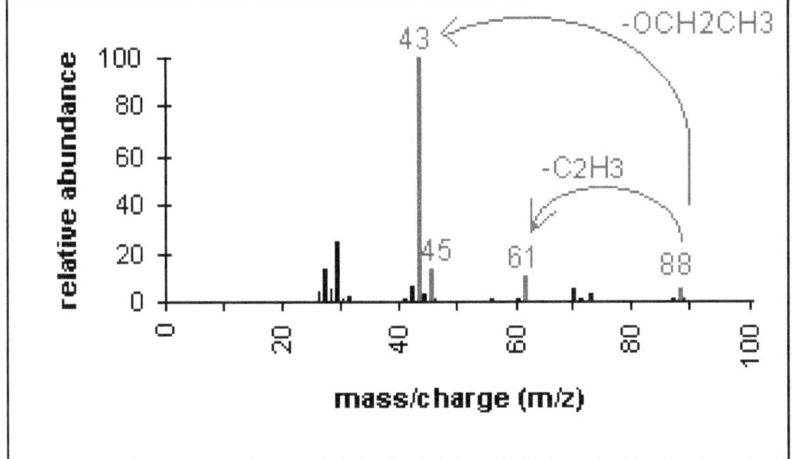

Figure 5.20 Mass spectrum of Ethyl acetate.

Ether

- Fragmentation tends to occur alpha to the oxygen atom (C-C bond next to the oxygen).
- Ethyl methyl ether (C_3H_8O) with MW = 60.10 (Figure 5.21)

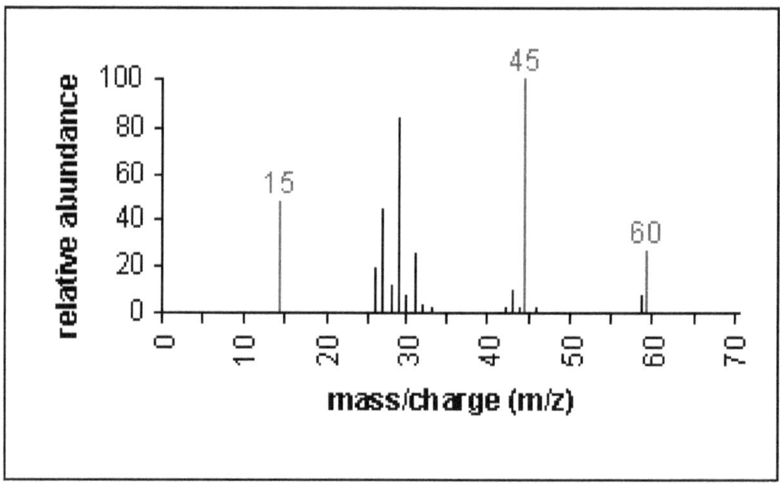

Figure 5.21 Mass spectrum of Ethyl methyl ether.

Halide

- The presence of chlorine or bromine atoms is usually recognizable from isotopic peaks.

- 1-Bromopropane (C_3H_7Br) with MW = 123.00 (Figure 5.22)

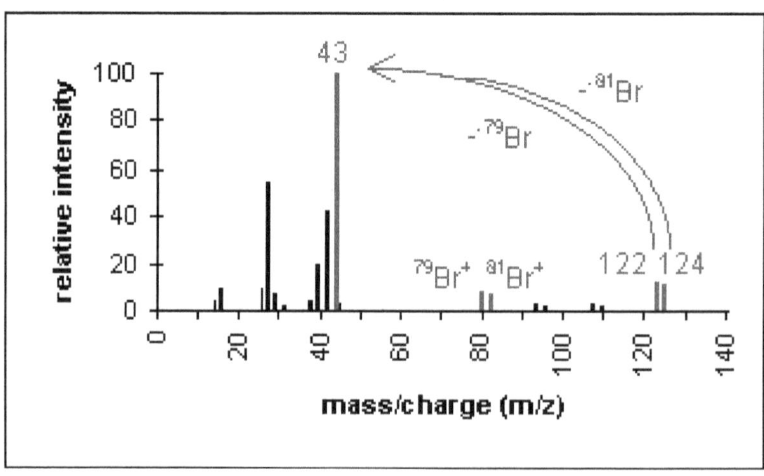

Figure 5.22 Mass spectrum of 1-Bromopropane.

Ketone

- Major fragmentation peaks result from cleavage of the C-C bonds adjacent to the carbonyl.

- 4-Heptanone ($C_7H_{14}O$) with MW = 114.19 (Figure 5.23)

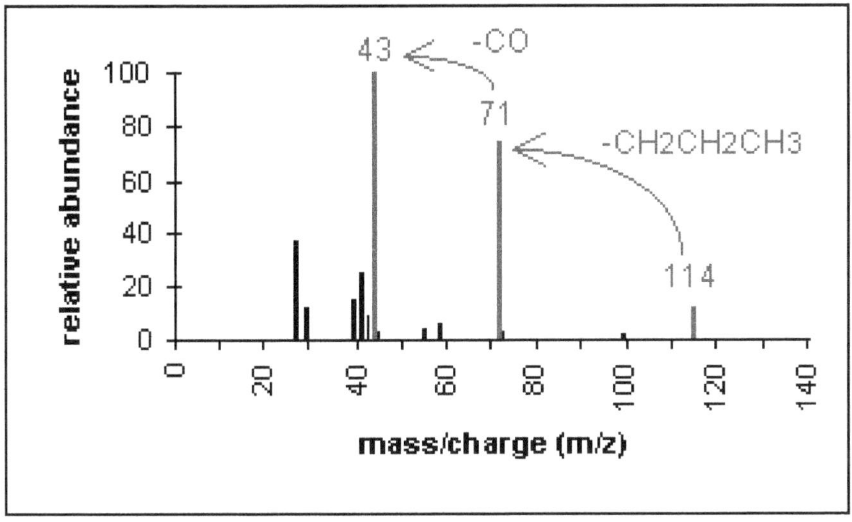

Figure 5.23 Mass spectrum of 4-Heptanone.

Rules in Mass Spectrometry

Nitrogen Rule

'The nitrogen rule states that organic molecules that contain hydrogen, carbon, nitrogen, oxygen, silicon, phosphorus, sulfur, and the halogens have an odd nominal mass if they have an odd number of nitrogen atoms or an even mass if they have an even number of nitrogen atoms are present'.

Table 5.1 Nitrogen rule

Even molecular weight	Nitrogen may be present or may not be present	Presence of Nitrogen in even number or Zero
Odd molecular weight	Molecule contain nitrogen	Presence odd nitrogen only CHNX)

Examples:

Table 5.2 Nitrogen rule - Example

Compound	Number of nitrogen	Molecular weight
H_2O	0 (No nitrogen)	18 (even)
CO_2	0 (No nitrogen)	44 (even)
NH_3	1 (odd nitrogen)	17 (odd)
NH_2-CO-NH_2 (urea)	2 (Even nitrogen)	60 (even)
NH_2OH	1 (odd nitrogen)	33 (odd)

Ring equivalence plus double bond equivalence or Index of Hydrogen deficiency:

The following formula from a molecular formula will give the information of number of ring / double bond in the structure.

$$\text{Rings} + \pi \text{ Bonds} = u = C - \frac{H}{2} - \frac{X}{2} + \frac{N}{2} + 1$$

Examples:

Table 5.3 Value of number of ring / double bond in the structure

Formula	u = value	Justification
CO2 (O=C=O)	2	The presence of two double bond in the structure
H2O (H-O-H)	0	No double bond or Ring
C6H6	4	the three double bond and one ring in Benzene

Even electron rule: The even electron rule states that ions with an even number of electrons (cations but not radical ions) tend to form even-electron fragment ions and odd-electron ions (radical ions) form odd-electron ions or even-electron ions Even-electron species tend to fragment to another even-electron cation and a neutral molecule rather than two odd-electron species.

Rule of 13

- The **Rule of 13** is used for tabulating possible chemical formula for a given molecular mass.

- It is based on the assumption that only carbon and hydrogen are present in the molecule , so the molecule comprises some number of CH "units"(has a nominal mass of 12+1 = 13).

- If the molecular weight of the molecule in question is M, the number of possible CH units is n and if r is the remainder

$$\frac{M}{13} = n + \frac{r}{13}$$

The base formula for the molecule is

$$C_nH_{n+r}$$

And the degree of unsaturation is

$$u = \frac{(n - r + 2)}{2}$$

Note: 'A negative value of u indicates the presence of heteroatoms in the molecule a half-integer value of u indicates the presence of an odd number of nitrogen atoms. On addition of heteroatoms, the molecular formula is adjusted by the equivalent mass of carbon and hydrogen. For example, adding N requires removing CH_2 and adding O requires removing CH_4'.

Stevenson's Rule

- Upon dissociation of AB+.→A++ B.or A+ B+A+will be formed if it has the lower ionization energy

- In branched radical cations, the largest group is preferentially lost

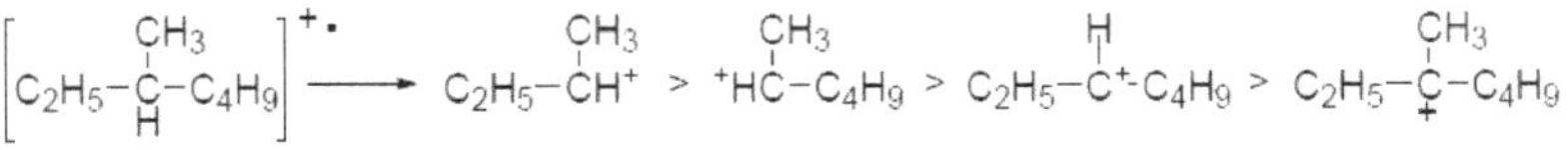

$$\left[C_2H_5 - \overset{\overset{\displaystyle CH_3}{|}}{\underset{\underset{\displaystyle H}{|}}{C}} - C_4H_9 \right]^{+\cdot} \longrightarrow C_2H_5 - \overset{\overset{\displaystyle CH_3}{|}}{C}H^+ \; > \; {}^+H\overset{\overset{\displaystyle CH_3}{|}}{C} - C_4H_9 \; > \; C_2H_5 - \overset{\overset{\displaystyle H}{|}}{C}{}^+ \text{-} C_4H_9 \; > \; C_2H_5 - \overset{\overset{\displaystyle CH_3}{|}}{\underset{\underset{\displaystyle +}{}}{C}} - C_4H_9$$

Fragmentation Rule

- The intensity of molecular ion is high for straight chain compounds.

- The fragmentation peak intensity will be high for branched compounds.

- Heterocyclic compounds (pyridine) undergo more fragmentation than carbocyclic compounds (benzene).

- Stability of alkene is favored by allylcation (+CH=CH- CH3), stability order is based on sayzteff rule.

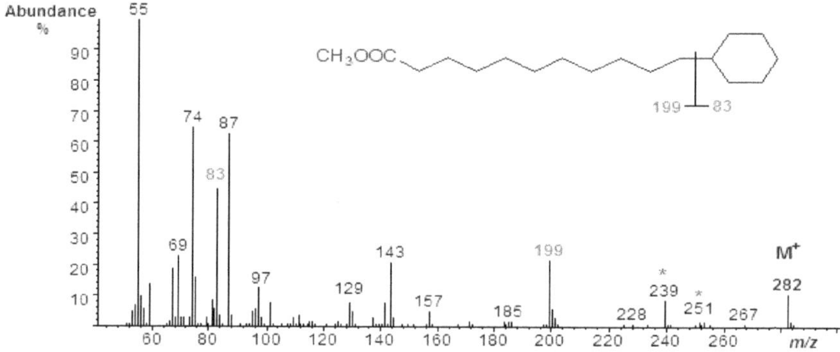

- Alpha cleavage is common with cycloalkane

Figure 5.24 Mass spectrum of cycloalkane.

- Beta cleavage is favored for alkyl benzene and followed by the formation of more stable tropilium ion

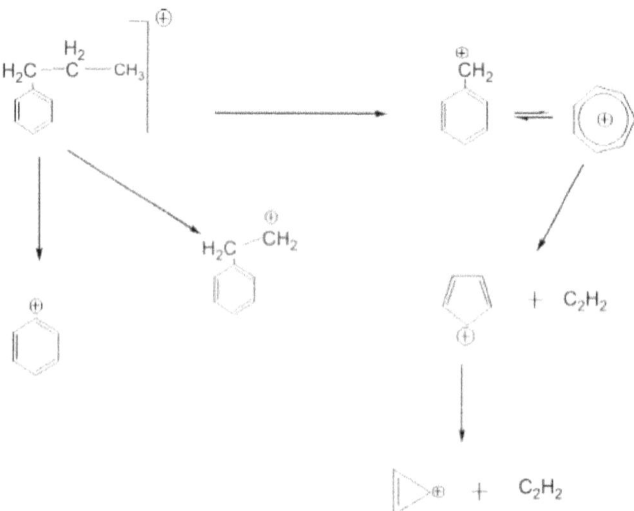

Figure 5.25 Beta-cleavage of tropilium ion.

Retro - Diels – Alder Reaction:

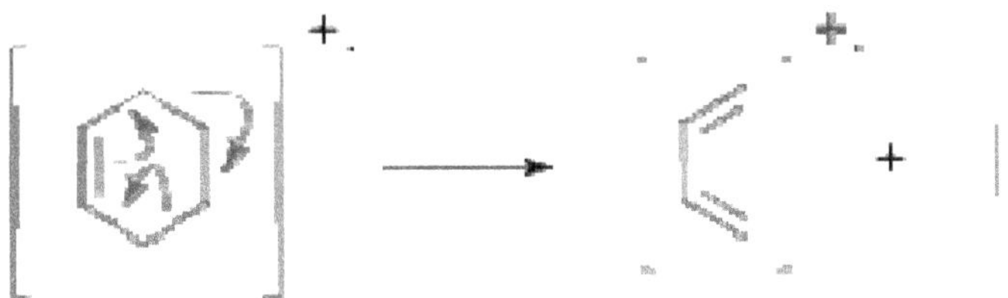

Mc- Lafferty rearrangement of Compounds contains gamma hydrogen to C=X system (X = O, N, S).

Figure 5.26 Mc- Lafferty rearrangement

In case of heteroatoms in a chain C-C to next heteroatom will be cleaved. Example: alcohol and amines.

2-propanol
MW = 60

molecular ion
(highly unstable)

'oxonium' ion
m/z = 45

Fragmentation of carbonyl compounds:

acyl radical
(not detected)

methyl cation
m/z = 15

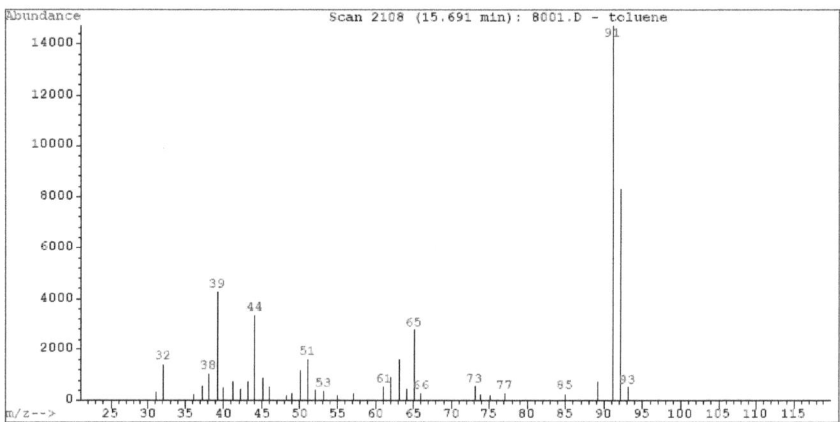

Exercise

Exercise 1: Identify the various peaks and predict the type of isotope based and abundance in the following spectrum?

Figure 5.27 Example spectrum for Exercise

Exercise 2: Identify the various ions in the given fragmentation pattern?

Exercise 3: Carry out fragmentation for the following structures ?

Chapter 6

Raman Spectroscopy

Raman spectroscopy based on Raman effect, in which beam of laser is passed through a sample and allowed for scattering. The scattered light is measure with respect to frequency. The Raman spectra are obtained using Raman shift (cm-1) and absorbance intensity in Y axis.

Raman spectroscopy based on the vibrational energy of the bond, and considered as complementary technique for IR absorption spectroscopy. The bonds which are IR inactive (example: H-H, N=N which dipole moment Zero), are active under Raman scattering. Because Raman absorption is depends on bond polarizability (selection and Mutual exclusion principle). The Phenomena of light interaction with matter shown in Figure 6.1 and Figure 6.2

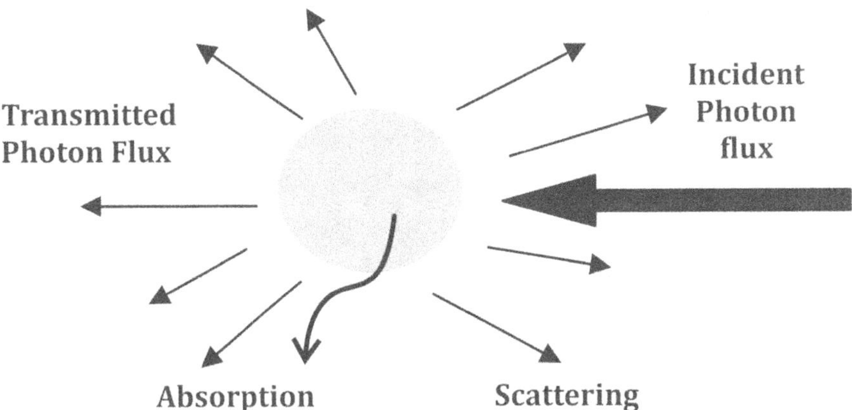

Figure 6.1 Interaction of light with matter.

Raman Shift

$$\Delta w = \left(\frac{1}{\lambda_0} - \frac{1}{\lambda_1} \right),$$

Where λ_0 is the wavelength of excitation light (incident) and λ_1 is the wavelength of Raman spectrum (scattered). There are three types of shift is observed (Figure 6.3).

1. Rayleigh (elastic) : λ_0 and λ_1 frequencies are equal

2. Stokes and anti-stokes (Raman inelastic):λ_0 and λ_1 are unequal as shown below.

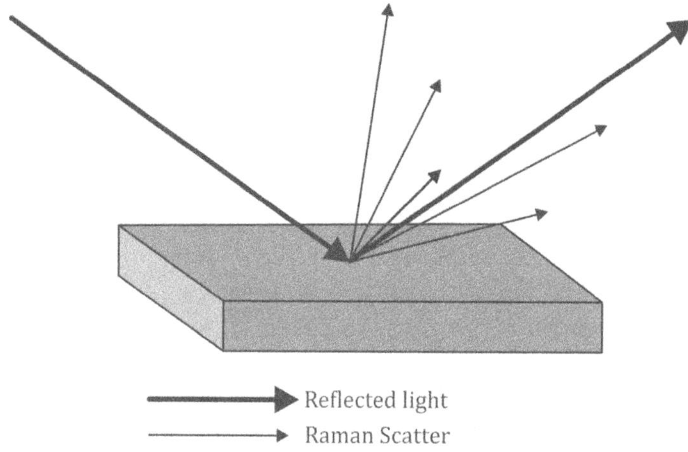

Figure 6.2 Raman effect – Reflected light (thin arrow) versus Raman Scatter (thick arrow).

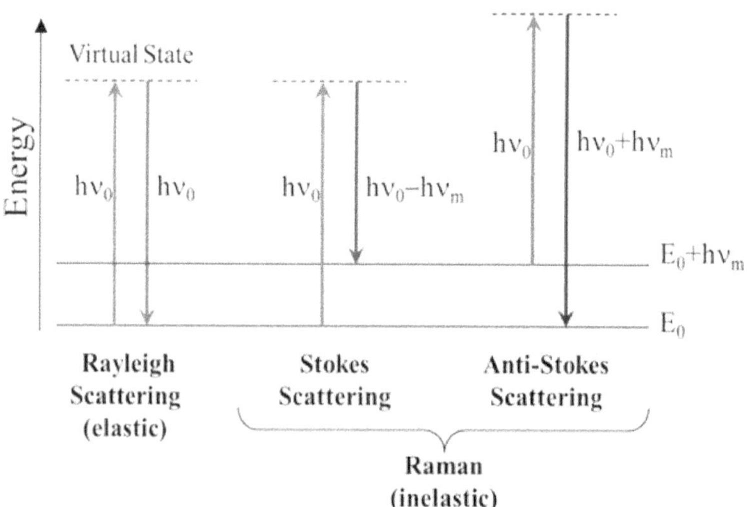

Figure 6.3 Raman Shift (Elastic and inelastic scattering).

A typical Raman Spectra is shown in Figure 6.4 (absorbance mode):

- The position of peaks are considered for qualitative information.

- The intensity is used for quantitative information regarding structure and its physico-chemical properties.
- The interpretation depends upon the sample's chemical nature, the probe range (Raman shift, cm-1).
- Specific vibration modes can be found for organic molecules. Fingerprint region for organic molecules ranges from 500cm-1 to 2000cm-1.
- If low frequency region is probed then crystal characteristics can be investigated as well.
- For finding the bond strength: its relatively easier for simple gas molecules like O2, N2 (rotation Raman lines).

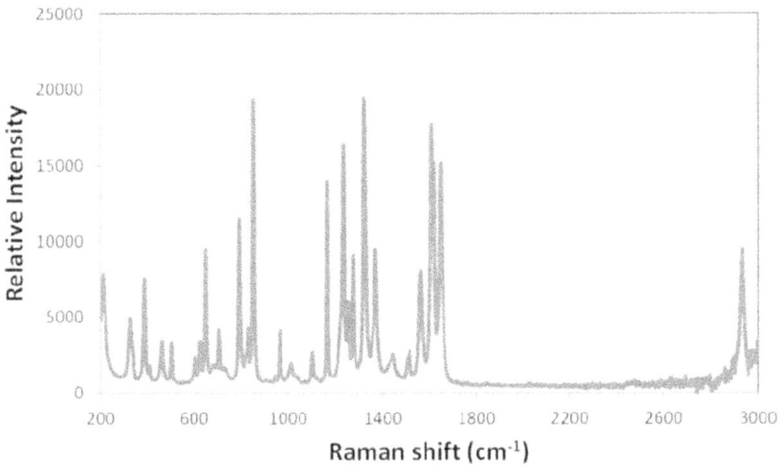

Figure 6.4 A typical Raman spectrum.

The following spectrum (Figure 6.5) showing the comparison of sorbic acid in solution form and crystal form

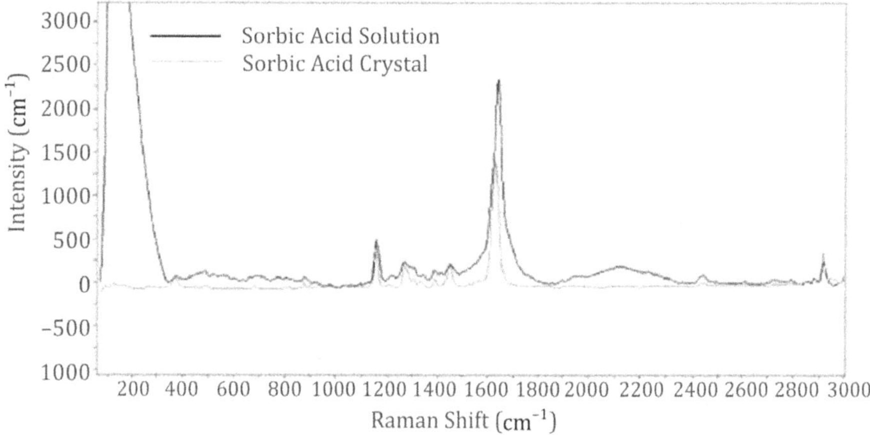

Figure 6.5 Raman spectra of sorbic acid solution vs sorbic acid solid (crystal).

Advantage of Raman Spectra

- Raman can be used to analyse aqueous solutions since it does not suffer from the large water absorption effects found with FT techniques.
- The intensity of spectral features in solution is directly proportional to the concentration of the particular species
- Raman spectra are generally robust to temperature changes
- Raman requires little or no sample preparation. It does not need the use of Nujol, or KBr matrices and is largely unaffected sample cell materials such as glass.
- The use of a Raman microscope provide very high level of spatial resolution and depth discrimination, not found with the FT methods of analysis

Disadvantage of Raman Spectroscopy

- The cost of required equipment has been the main obstacle to the widespread adaption of Raman spectroscopy for routine analysis;
- A major problem for Raman measurements lies in the high levels of fluorescence (intrinsic or caused by impurities) overlaying the Raman bands. However, in most cases, this can be avoided by shifting the laser wavelength to the NIR spectral region; and,
- If excitation intensities are too high, they may thermally decompose the sample.

Various Raman absorption characteristics for functional residue of structures: The frequencies are shown in table 6.1

Table 6.1 Various Raman and infrared absorption characteristics for functional residue of structures

Functional Group/ Vibration	Region	Raman	InfraRed
Lattice vibrations in crystals, LA modes	10 - 200 cm^{-1}	strong	strong
δ(CC) aliphatic chains	250 - 400 cm^{-1}	strong	weak
υ(Se-Se)	290 -330 cm^{-1}	strong	weak
υ(S-S)	430 -550 cm^{-1}	strong	weak
υ(Si-O-Si)	450 -550 cm^{-1}	strong	weak
υ(Xmetal-O)	150-450 cm^{-1}	strong	med-weak
υ(C-I)	480 - 660 cm^{-1}	strong	strong
υ(C-Br)	500 - 700 cm^{-1}	strong	strong
υ(C-Cl)	550 - 800 cm^{-1}	strong	strong
υ(C-S) aliphatic	630 - 790 cm^{-1}	strong	medium
υ(C-S) aromatic	1080 - 1100 cm^{-1}	strong	medium
υ(O-O)	845 -900 cm^{-1}	strong	weak
υ(C-O-C)	800 -970 cm^{-1}	medium	weak
υ(C-O-C) asym	1060 - 1150 cm^{-1}	weak	strong
υ(CC) alicyclic, aliphatic chain vibrations	600 - 1300 cm^{-1}	medium	Medium
υ(C=S)	1000 - 1250 cm^{-1}	strong	weak
υ(CC) aromatic ring chain vibrations	*1580, 1600 cm^{-1}	strong	medium
	*1450, 1500 cm^{-1}	medium	medium
	*1000 cm^{-1}	strong/medium	weak
δ(CH3)	1380 cm^{-1}	medium	strong
δ(CH2) δ(CH3) asym	1400 - 1470 cm^{-1}	medium	medium
δ(CH2) δ(CH3) asym	1400 - 1470 cm^{-1}	medium	medium
υ(C-(NO2))	1340 - 1380 cm^{-1}	strong	medium
υ(C-(NO2)) asym	1530 - 1590 cm^{-1}	medium	strong
υ(N=N) aromatic	1410 - 1440 cm^{-1}	medium	-
υ(N=N) aliphatic	1550 - 1580 cm^{-1}	medium	-
δ(H2O)	~1640 cm^{-1}	weak broad	strong
υ(C=N)	1610 - 1680 cm^{-1}	strong	medium
υ(C=C)	1500 - 1900 cm^{-1}	strong	weak
υ(C=O)	1680 - 1820 cm^{-1}	medium	strong
υ(C≅C)	2100 - 2250 cm^{-1}	strong	weak
υ(C≅N)	2220 - 2255 cm^{-1}	medium	strong
υ(-S-H)	2550 - 2600 cm^{-1}	strong	weak
υ(C-H)	2800 - 3000 cm^{-1}	strong	strong
υ(=(C-H))	3000 - 3100 cm^{-1}	strong	medium
υ(≅(C-H))	3300 cm^{-1}	weak	strong
υ(N-H)	3300 - 3500 cm^{-1}	medium	medium
υ(O-H)	3100 - 3650 cm^{-1}	weak	strong

Identification Compounds by Raman Spectra

The following Raman spectrum shows the identification of various nitrogen compounds. Raman spectral bands vary from one compound to another compound (Figure 6.6).

The following spectrum (Figure 6.7) shows the Raman spectra for different drug, in which Asprin and acetaminophen has structure resemblance of benzene derivatives. The bottom spectra is for caffeine, entirely different than above two spectra

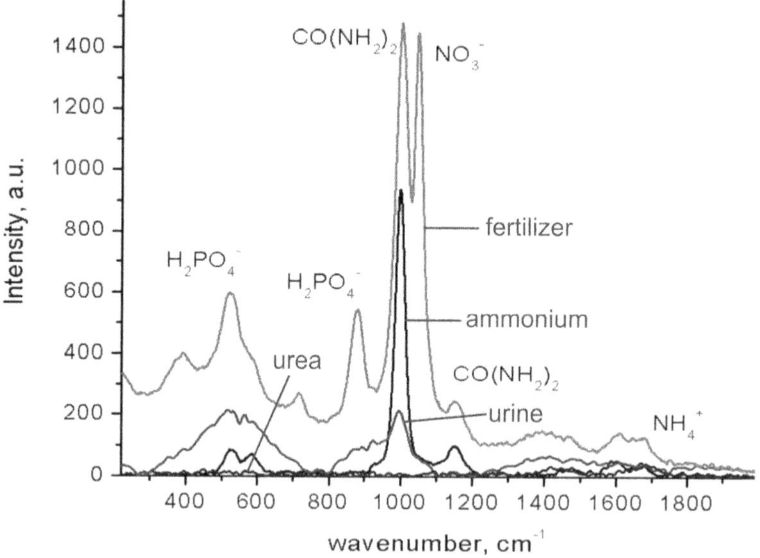

Figure 6.6 Identification of Nitrogen compounds by Raman Spectra.

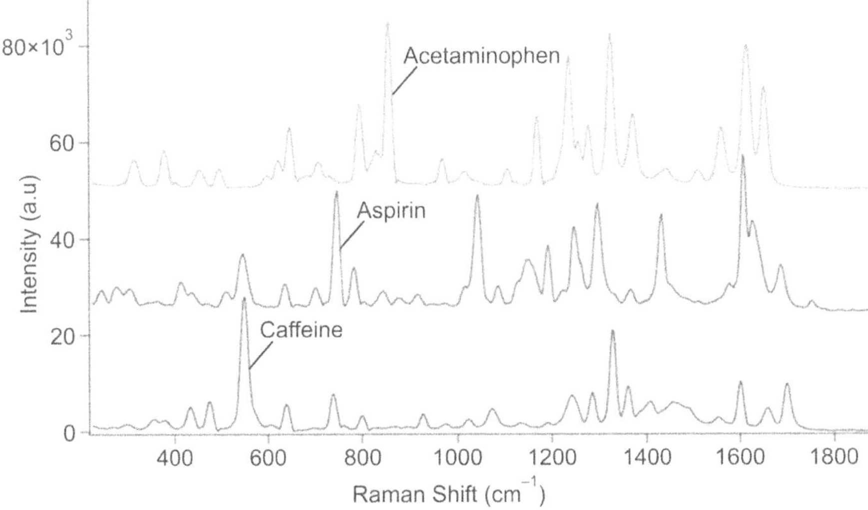

Figure 6.7 Raman spectra of Acetaminophen, Aspirin and Caffeine.

Identification of various inorganic elements by Raman spectra: Position of Raman shift vary from element to element, and the particular wavelength is used for identification of elements (Figure 6.8).

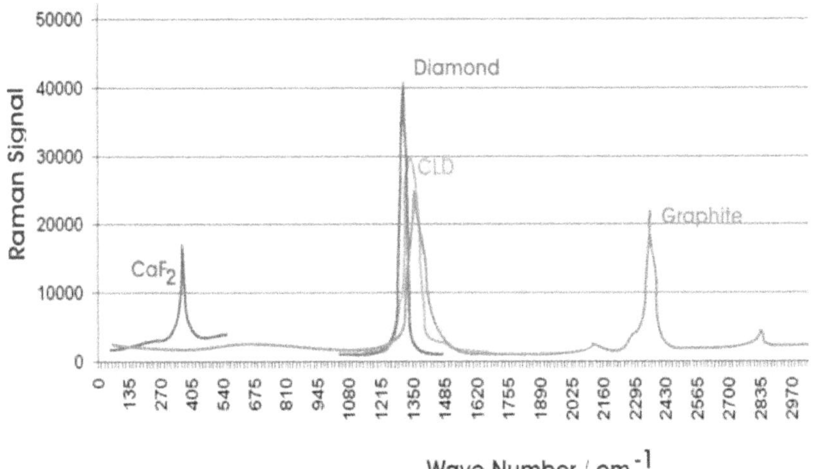

Figure 6.8 Raman spectra of Inorganic elements (diamond, Graphite and Calcium Fluride).

Example of Raman Spectra for Drugs

The following spectrum shows the Raman spectrum of paracetamol drug. And indicated the effect of measurement count with low' and without low'.

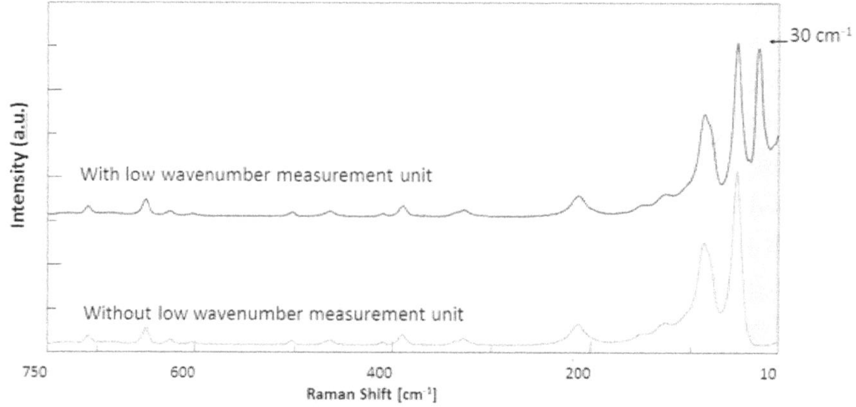

Figure 6.9 Raman spectrum of Paracetamol.

Raman Spectra in Identification of Metabolic Sites

Raman spectrum of Erlotinib measured in cells as compared to the free-Erlotinib spectrum indicate that Erlotinib is metabolized within cells to its demethylated derivative (Figure 6.10).

Raman Spectra in differentiation of Co-crystal and Mixture: The following spectrum (Figure 6.11) shows the difference between caffeine co-crystals with 2- benzoic acid and mixture of these two. The spectral characteristics were different for both.

Detection of Physical state of Ibuprofen in Solid dispersion: The following spectrum shows (Figure 6.12) Raman spectra for Ibuprofen (a) hydrate isomalt (b) de-hydrated isomalt (c). The Intensity at 874 783, 746 cm-1 were considered as indicator wavenumber to assess the physical state of active ingredient in formulations.

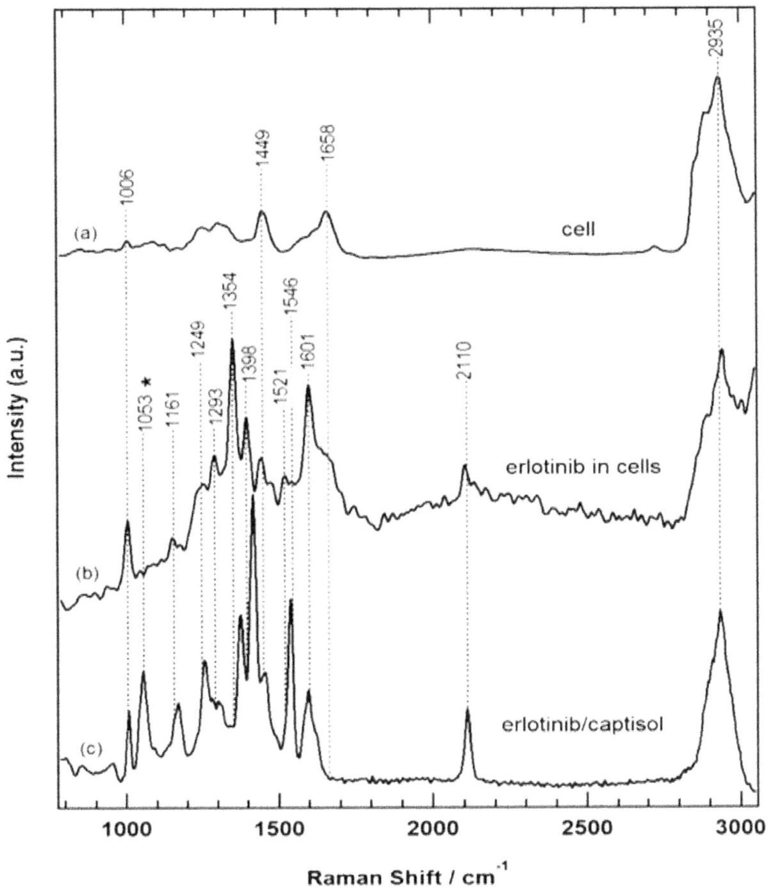

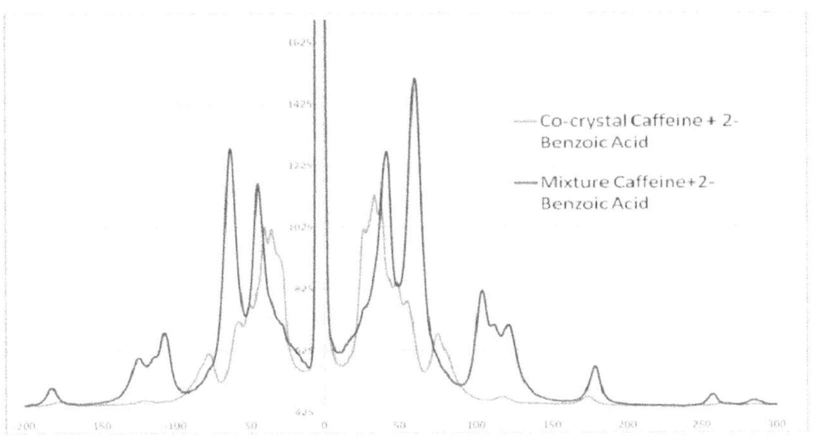

Figure 6.10 Overlay Raman spectra of Erlotinib.

Figure 6.11 Raman spectra of caffeine with 2- benzoic acid.

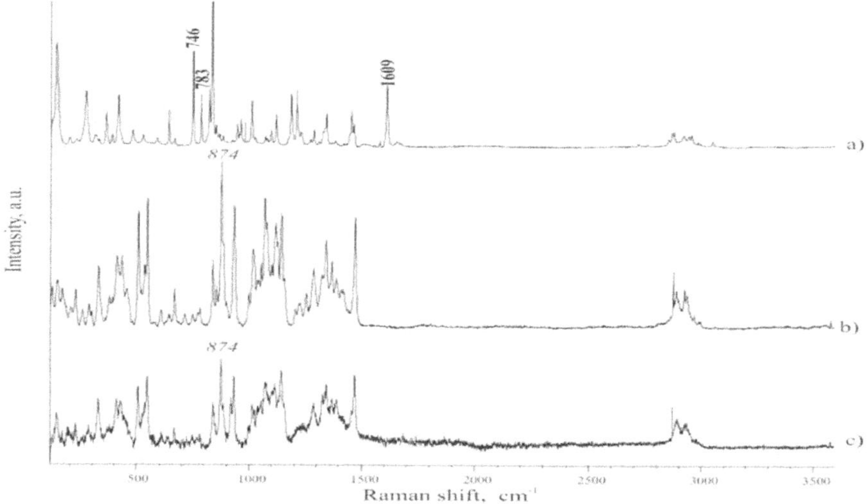

Figure 6.12 Raman spectra of Ibuprofen.

Polymorph study: Differentiation of anhydrous and hydrate form of Pharmaceuticals: There two examples has been given for the polymorph of Theophylline (Figure 6.13) and different hexoses (Figure 6.14).

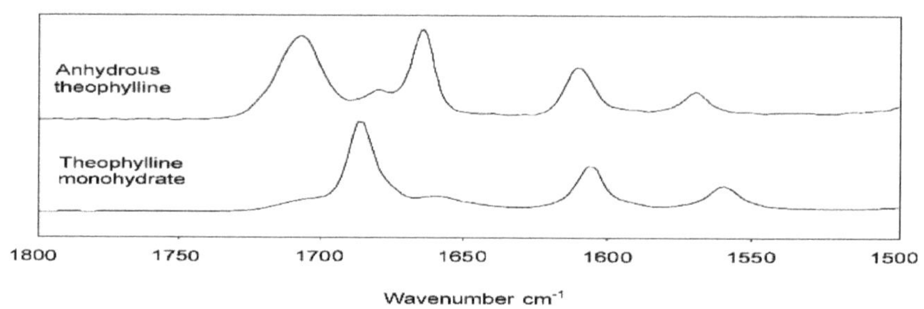

Figure 6.13 Raman spectra of Polymorph of Theophylline.

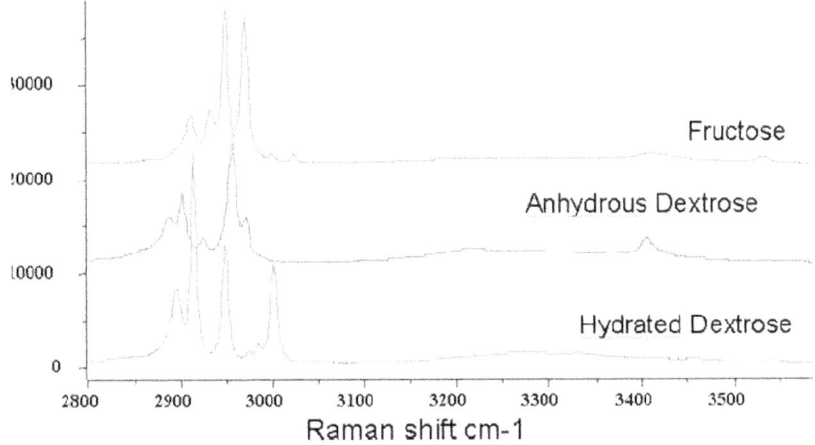

Figure 6.14 Raman spectra of different hexoses.

The following spectrum shows (Figure 6.15) the two different form of stearic acid while precipitated in hexane.

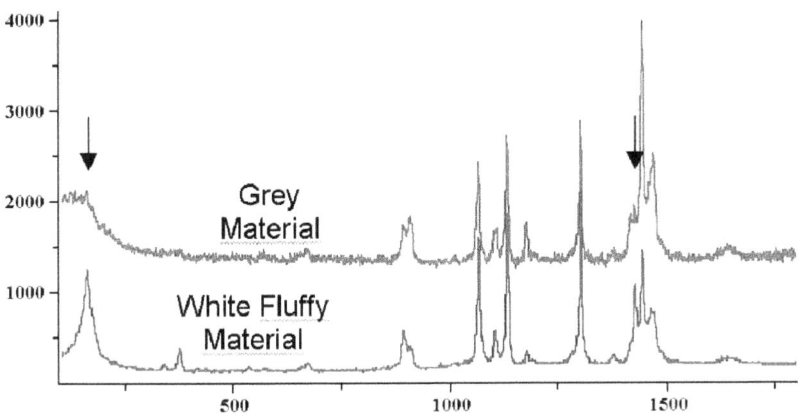

Figure 6.15 Raman spectra of stearic acid in hexane.

Example Raman spectra of IA, IB and form II exhibit characteristic peaks that allow the identification of the polymorphic form. The differing features include form II peaks at 1305.7 cm^{-1}, 1185 cm^{-1} 1247 cm^{-1}, and form I peaks at 1208 cm^{-1} and 1120 - 1140 cm^{-1}. When the spectra were overlaid the form I peak at 1208 cm^{-1} and the form II peak at 1185cm^{-1} were judged most suitable for identification. These peaks also offer potential for a quantitative analysis of polymorphic mixtures (Figure 6.16).

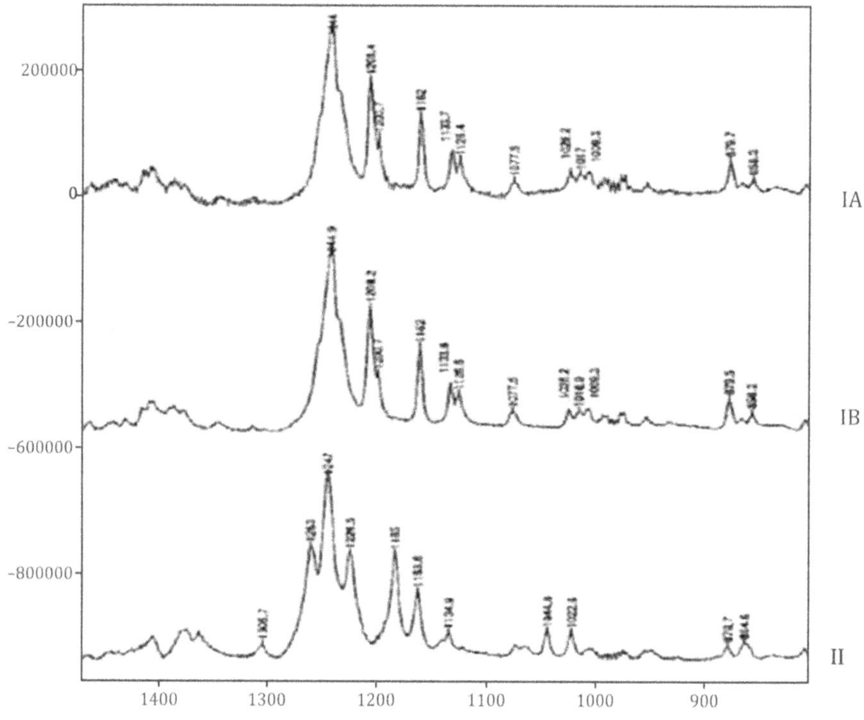

Figure 6.16 Identification of Polymorphs by Raman spectra.

Differentiation of different crystalline nature of Pharmaceutical substance: As crystalline nature increases the intensity increases. Note that there is no change in Raman shift (Figure 6.17).

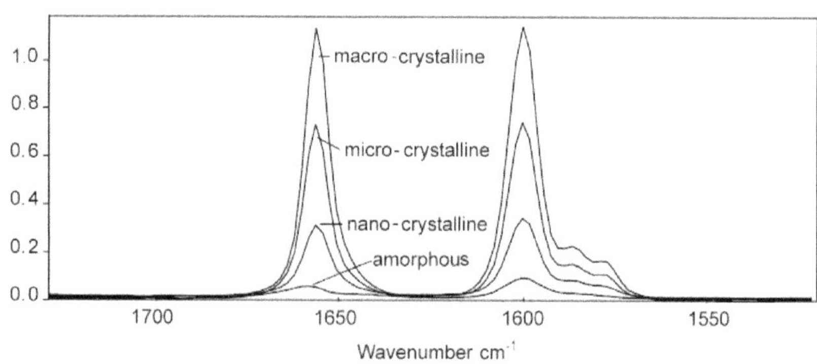

Figure 6.17 Differentiation of different crystalline nature by Raman spectra.

Characterization and Mapping of active pharmaceutical ingredients and excipients in a tablet Raman Spectroscopy: The following spectrum shows (Figure 6.18) the tablet of same drug in two different diluent viz starch (a) and lactose (b), which can be used as standard to identify the formulation.

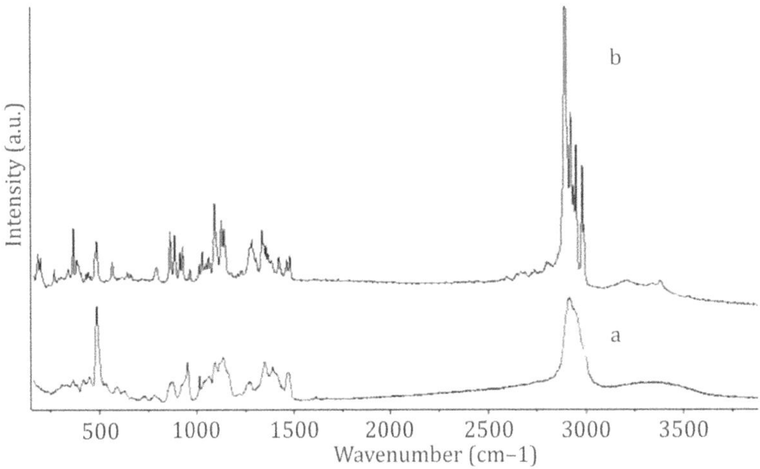

Figure 6.18 Characterization and Mapping of active pharmaceutical ingredients and excipients in a tablet.

Raman spectroscopy in tablet coating: Raman spectroscopy for the determination of coating uniformity of tablets: The quality, stability, safety, and performance of the final product depend largely on the amount and uniformity of coating applied. The bottom most spectrum is core tablet. Middle spectrum is for coated tablet. Upper one is spectrum for coating material (Figure 6.19).

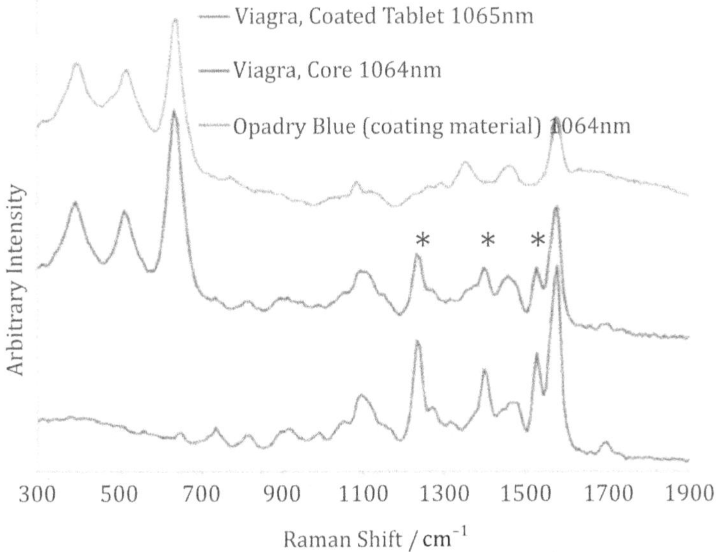

Figure 6.19 Raman spectra in tablet coating (* coated tablet).

Physical stability and recrystallization kinetics of amorphous drug product by Raman spectroscopy: The solid-state physical stability and recrystallization kinetics during storage for an amorphous solid dispersed drug substance can be carried out by using Raman spectroscopy. In the spectra A is pure, B, C are degraded substance (Figure 6.20).

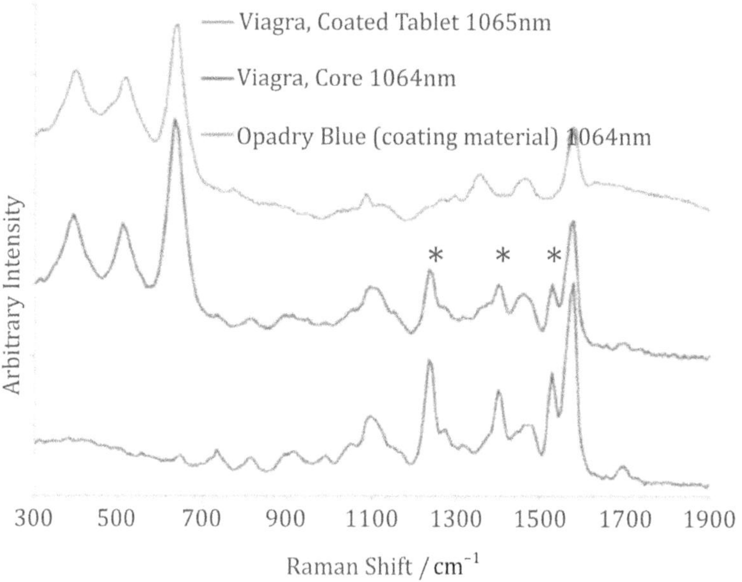

Figure 6.20 Raman spectra in Physical stability of a drug.

Thermal Methods of Analysis

Thermal analysis is a branch of materials science where the properties of materials (drugs) are studied as they change with temperature.

Types of Thermal Methods of Analysis

Table 6.2 Types of thermal methods

Dielectric thermal analysis (DEA): dielectric permittivity and loss factor
Differential thermal analysis (DTA): temperature difference verus temperature or time
Differential Scanning Calorimetry (DSC): heat flow changes versus temperature or time
Dilatometry (DIL): volume changes with temperature change

Table 6.2 *contd...*

Dynamic Mechanical Analysis (DMA or DMTA) : measures storage modulus (stiffness) and loss modulus (damping) versus temperature, time and frequency
Evolved Gas Analysis (EGA) : analysis of gases evolved during heating of a material, usually decomposition products
Laser flash analysis (LFA): thermal diffusivity and thermal conductivity
Thermogravimetric Analysis (TGA): mass change versus temperature or time
Thermomechanical analysis (TMA): dimensional changes versus temperature or time
Thermo-optical analysis (TOA): optical properties
Derivatography: A complex method in thermal analysis
Simultaneous Thermal Analysis (STA) generally refers to the simultaneous application of Thermogravimetry (TGA)

DSC and TGA test conditions are perfectly identical (same atmosphere, gas flow rate, vapor pressure of the sample, heating rate, thermal contact to the sample crucible and sensor, radiation effect, etc.). But they differ in output measurement. Energy is measured in DSC where as temperature difference measured in TGA. The information gathered can even be enhanced by coupling the STA instrument to an Evolved Gas Analyzer (EGA) like Fourier transform infrared spectroscopy (FTIR) or mass spectrometry (MS). The essence of all these techniques is that the sample's response is recorded as a function of temperature (and time), which is defined as "thermogram". Measurements may be carried out in air or under an inert gas (e.g. nitrogen or helium).

NOTE: Inverse gas chromatography is a technique depends on interaction between gases and vapours (surface – measurements) often made at different temperatures. Hence this technique also classified as thermal Analysis.

Chapter 7

Differential Scanning Calorimetry (DSC)

Differential scanning calorimetry (DSC), is a thermoanalytical or thermal method of analysis, where the difference in the amount of heat in the form of energy is measured between sample (analyte) and reference, as a function of temperature, while both analyte and reference are at the same temperature throughout the experiment (Figure 7.1). The temperature program in DSC analysis is designed as temperature increases linearly as a function of time. The reference sample (eg. Alumina) should have a well-defined **heat capacity** over the range of temperatures to be scanned

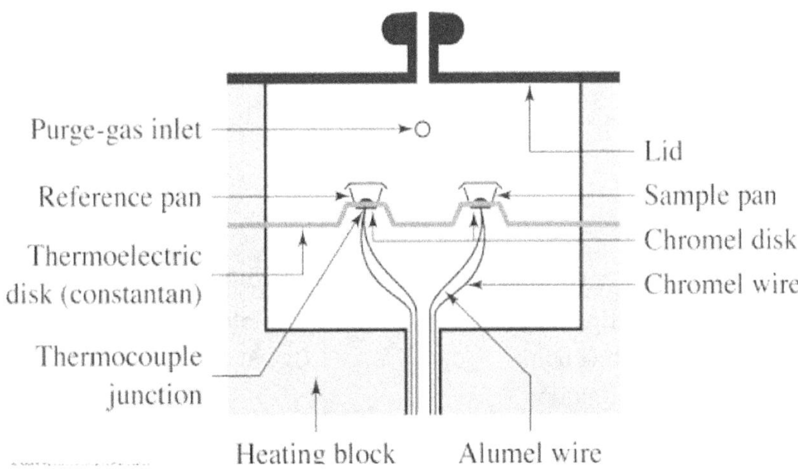

Figure 7.1 Differential scanning calorimeter (DSC).

DSC Curves or Thermogram

DSC curve (Figure 7.2) is drawn heat flux versus temperature or versus time. There are two different conventions: exothermic reactions in the sample shown with a positive or negative peak, depending on the kind of technology used in the experiment. This curve can be used to calculate enthalpies of transitions. This is done by integrating the peak corresponding to a given transition using the equation

$\Delta H = KA$

ΔH = Enthalpy, K = Calorimetric constant, A = area of the peak

Qualitative Approach of DSC Thermogram

There are various physiochemical changes take place when a substance is exposed to temperature programme. The important changes are shown in below diagram (Figure 7.2).

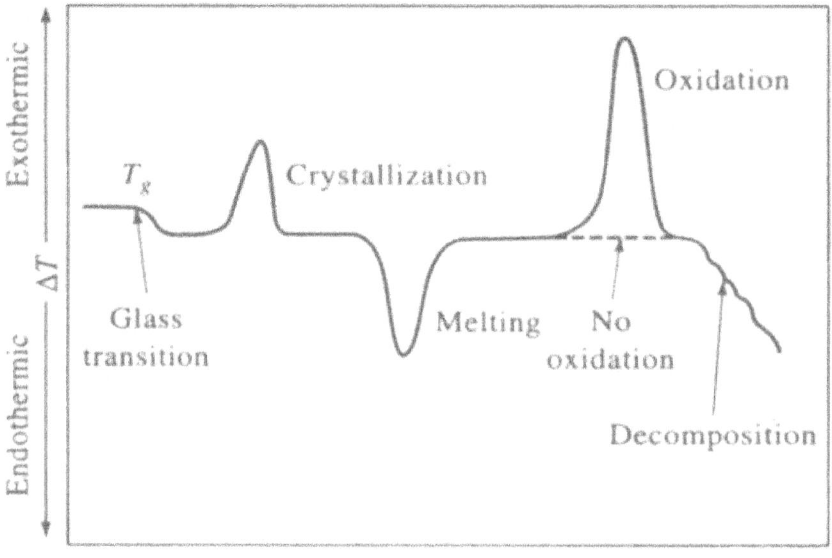

Endothermic	Exothermic
Melting point	Crystallization
Boiling point	Oxidation
Sublimation	
Vaporization	
Desolvation	
Solid-solid phase transition	
Chemical degradation	

Figure 7.2 DSC thermogram.

Application of DSC in Pharmaceuticals

1. To determine the purity of a sample

2. To determine the number of polymorphs and to determine the ratio of each polymorph.

3. To determine the heat of salvation.

4. To determine the thermal degradation of a drug or excipients.

5. To determine the glass-transition temperature (tg) of a polymer.

Parameter to be considered in Interpretation of DSC

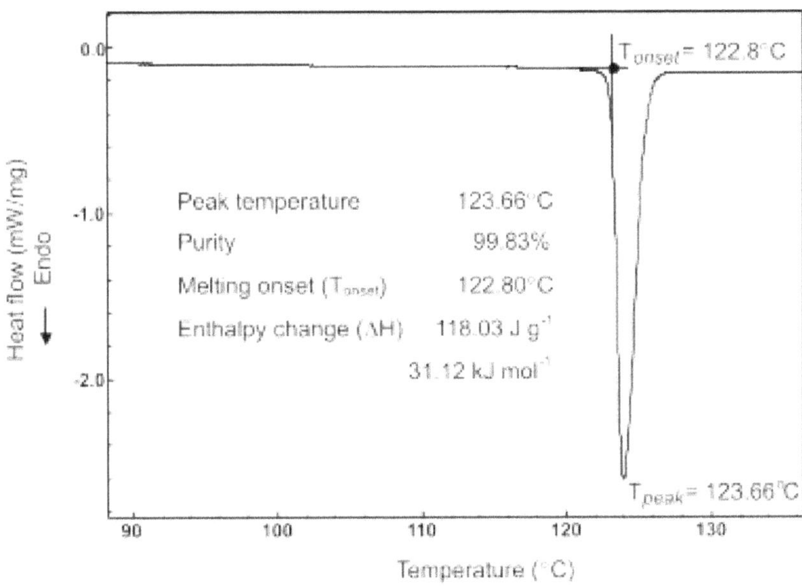

Figure 7.3 Interpretation of DSC thermogram.

There are four important parameters has been observed while interpreting the DSC

1. T max or T peak - Peak temperature (Physical and Chemical interaction, polymorphism).

2. T onset (for presence of impurity / drug load / physical interaction, polymorphism)

3. Area (Purity or quantification)

4. Enthalpy (quatification, impurity, purity, crystalline nature) (Figure 7.3).

Quantification by DSC

Quantification is done based on enthalpy, peak area measurement in which peak area is directly proportional to amount. The figure shown below (Figure 7.4) is the relationship between, amount of substance, peak area and enthalpy.

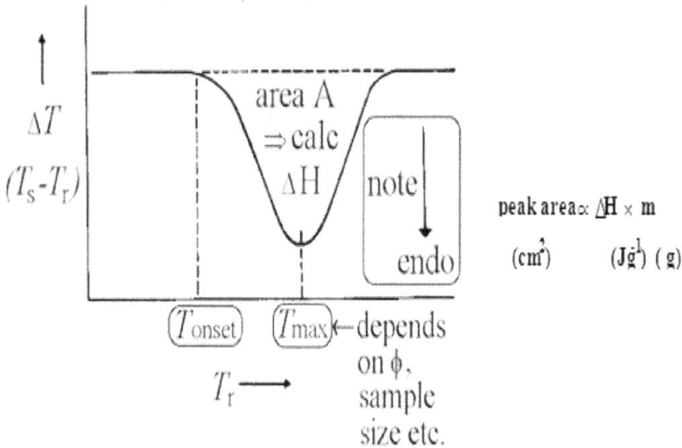

Figure 7.4 Quantification by DSC.

Identification Stereoisomers

The following thermogram shows (Figure 7.5) the characteristic difference between R, S, RS form of Omeprazole. They differ in shape, onset and T max of exothermic peak.

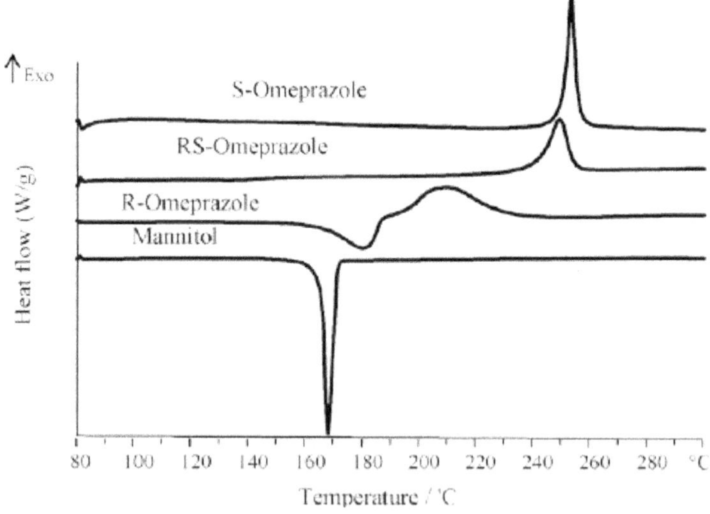

Figure 7.5 Identification of stereo-isomers by DSC thermogram.

Identification of Drugs

Below DSC thermogram, shows that five different drugs that they differ in melting point peak (endothermic peak) at 141 $^{\circ}$C, 174 $^{\circ}$C, 190 $^{\circ}$C, 200 $^{\circ}$C, 295 $^{\circ}$C. The same concept may be applied to differentiate polymers with alkyl derivatives, like methyl cellulose and ethyl cellulose (Figure 7.6).

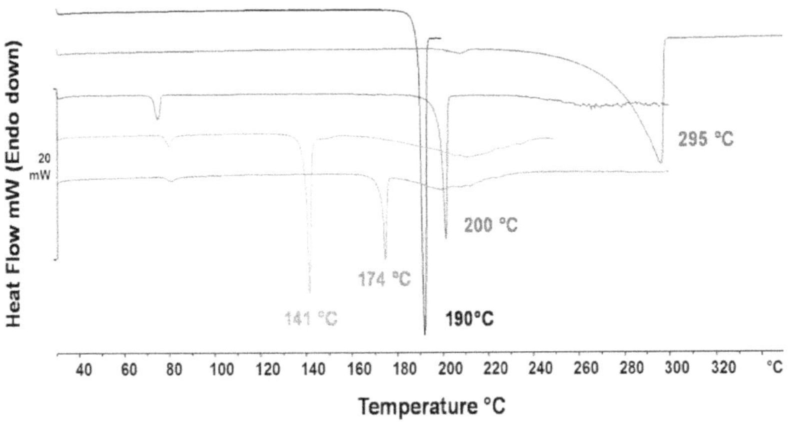

Figure 7.6 Melting points of different drugs by DSC thermogram.

Drug – Excipient Compatibility Studies

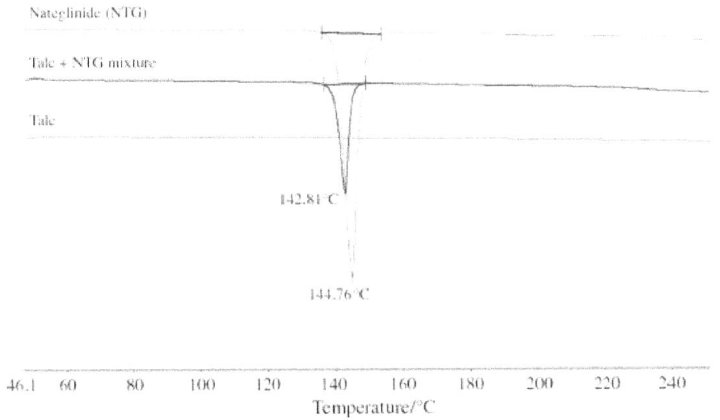

Figure 7.7 Drug – excipient compatibility studies by DSC.

The below DSC thermogram shows the compatibility of nateglinide drug with Talc. The melting point peak of 144 $^{\circ}$C (natiglinide) did not show significant shift in presence of talc (142 $^{\circ}$C). The shift of 2-5 $^{\circ}$C is quite acceptable; it is due the impurity effect, when combined with talc. The chemical interaction always shows significant shift of melting point and change in peak shape as well. Below is the another example where Nateglinide is compatible with Lactose (Figure 7.8).

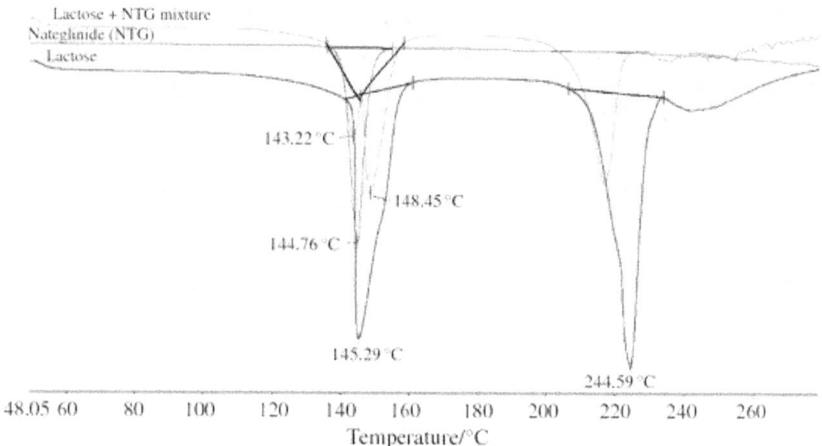

Figure 7.8 DSC thermogram - Compatibility of drug with excipients.

Detection of enantiotropic polymorphic conversion

The below thermogram shows (Figure 7.9) the enantiotropic polymorphic of drug Form I to Form II, after recrystallization. This is the one of the important behavior of drug molecule, which may affect dissolution.

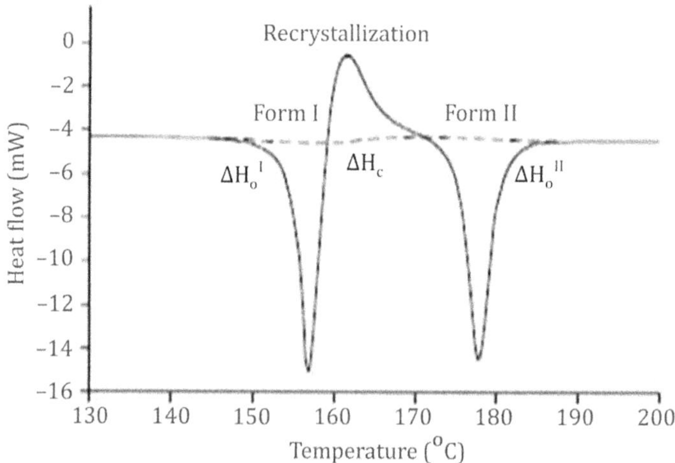

Figure 7.9 Detection of enantiotropic polymorphic conversion by DSC.

Detection of Pseudopolymorphism

Pseudopolymorphism is due the hydration or salvation. The below thermogram shows (Figure 7.10) the Pseudopolymorphism of hydrated glucose which shows two endothermic peaks along with shift of melting point of 5-10 °C.

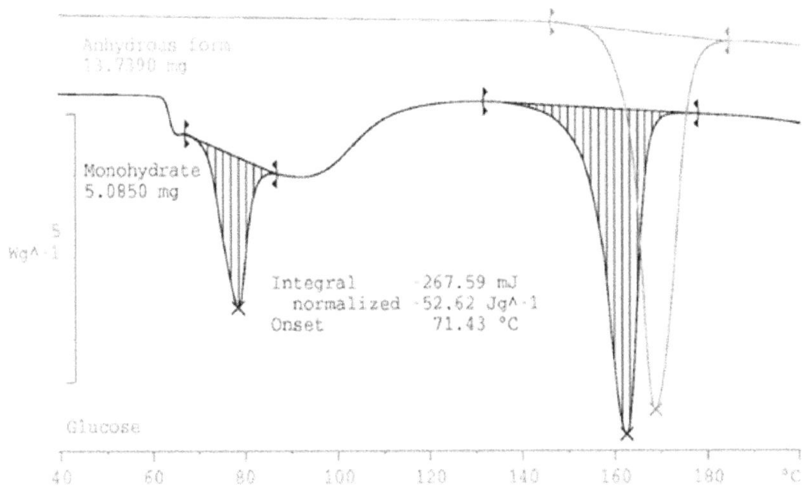

Figure 7.10 Detection of Pseudopolymorphism by DSC.

Study of Inclusion Complex

Cyclodextrin (CD) is the best example for excipient that form inclusion complex with drugs. The below thermogram shown (Figure 7.11) the successful formulation of inclusion complex shows the definite shift of melting point to lower temperature with broad peak shape. The below thermogram also indicated that physical mixture of estradiol and CD not suitable for formation of inclusion complex.

The below thermogram (Figure 7.12) is the example of inclusion complex between Furosemide and Cyclodextrin.

Detection of Drug Load in Microsphere

The below thermogram shows (Figure 7.13) the vancomycin loaded microsphere, where the slight elevation was noticed as compared to unloaded microsphere.

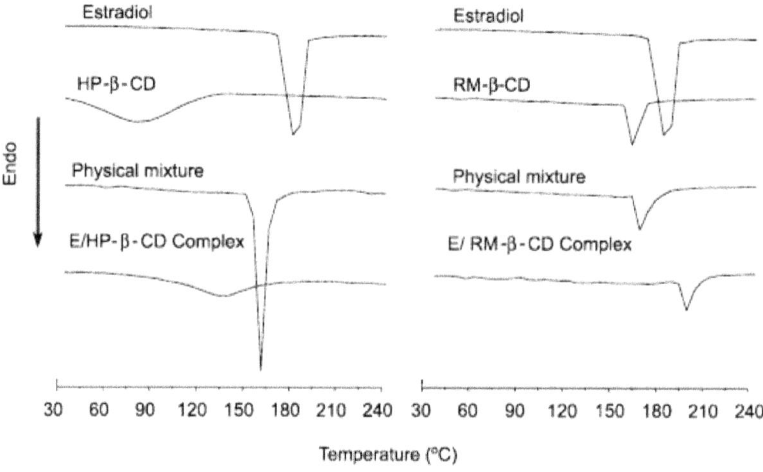

Figure 7.11 DSC thermogram of Cyclodextrin inclusion complex with Estradiol.

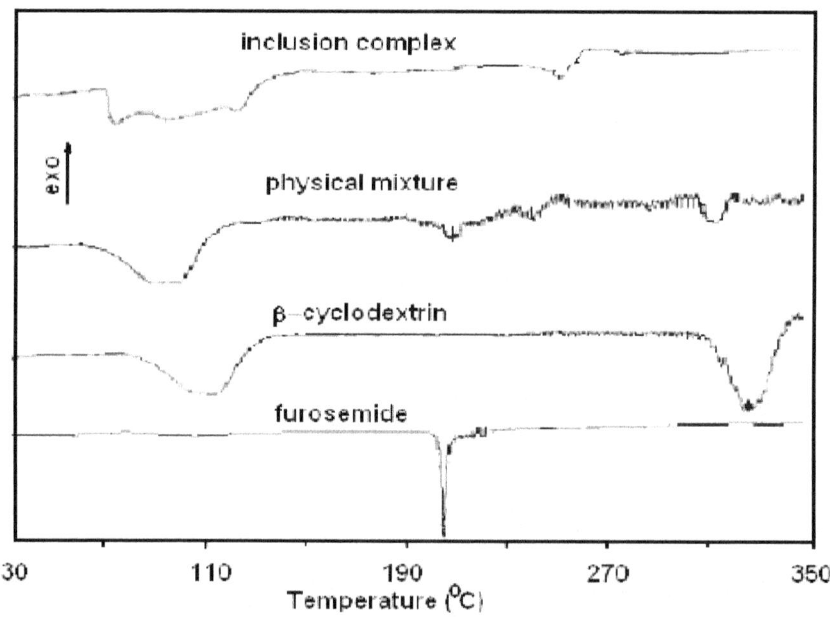

Figure 7.12 DSC thermogram of Cyclodextrin inclusion complex with Furosemide.

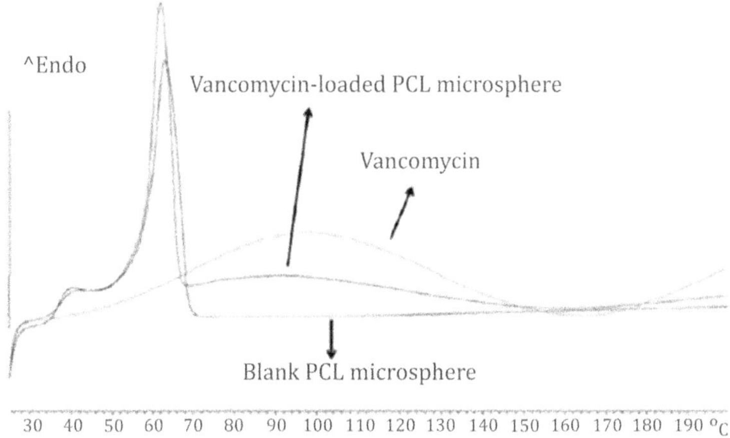

Figure 7.13 DSC thermogram of vancomycin loaded microsphere compared to unloaded microsphere.

Detection of Drug Load in Liposome

The change in shape and onset of endothermic peak at 110 ^{O}C indicated the drug load in Liposomes (Figure 7.14).

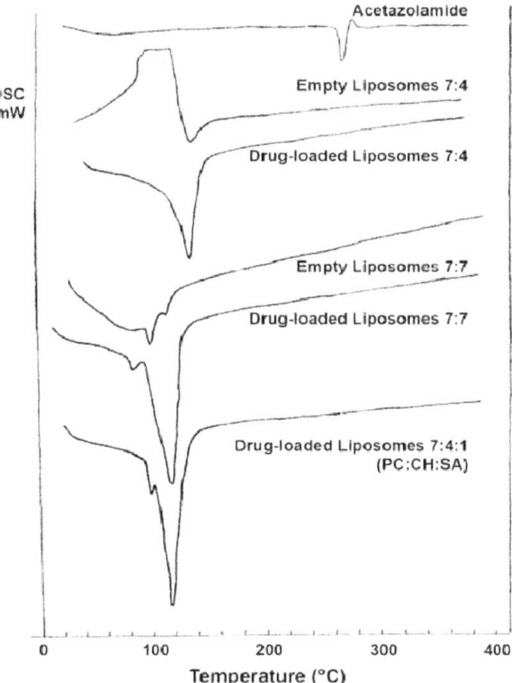

Figure 7.14 Detection of drug load in liposome by DSC.

Chapter 8

X-ray Diffraction Studies

X-rays

X-radiation (composed of **X-rays**) is a form of electromagnetic radiation. Most X-rays have a **wavelength** ranging from 0.01 to 10 nanometers, corresponding to frequencies in the range 30 **petahertz** to 30 **exahertz** (3×10^{16} Hz to 3×10^{19} Hz) and energies in the range 100 **eV** to 100 **keV**. X-ray wavelengths are shorter than those of <u>UV</u> rays and typically longer than those of **gamma rays**. In many languages, X-radiation is referred to with terms meaning **Roentgen radiation**,

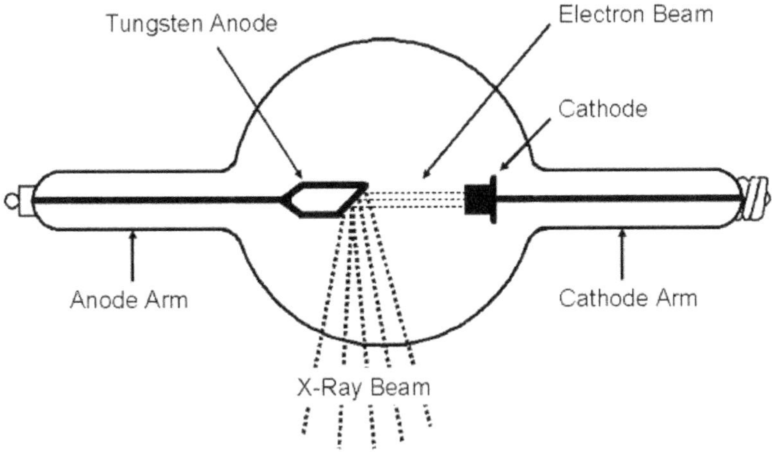

Figure 8.1 X-ray production (X-ray tube or Coolidge tube).

Production

X-rays can be generated by an **X-ray tube**, a **vacuum tube** that uses a high voltage to accelerate the **electrons** released by a **hot cathode** to a high velocity. The high velocity electrons collide with a metal target, the **anode**, creating the X-rays. In medical X-ray tubes the target is usually **tungsten** or a more crack-resistant alloy of **rhenium** (5%) and tungsten (95%), but sometimes **molybdenum** for more specialized applications, such as when softer X-rays are needed as in mammography. In crystallography, a **copper** target is most common, with **cobalt** often being used when fluorescence from **iron** content in the sample might otherwise present a problem (Figure 8.1).

There are two types of X-rays produced K-alpha and K-beta. K indicate the electron evalucated by electron beam. Alpha indicate L shell electron shift to K shell. Beta indicates the M shell electron shift to K shell. K- alpha more intense with longer wavelength than K beta (Figure 8.2).

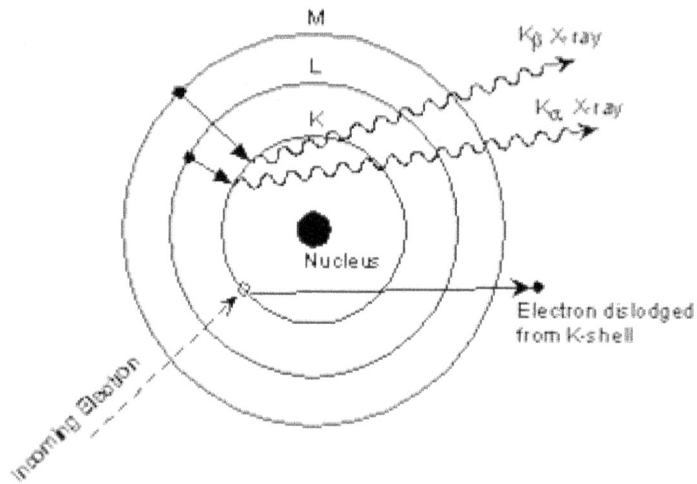

Figure 8.2 Types of X-rays.

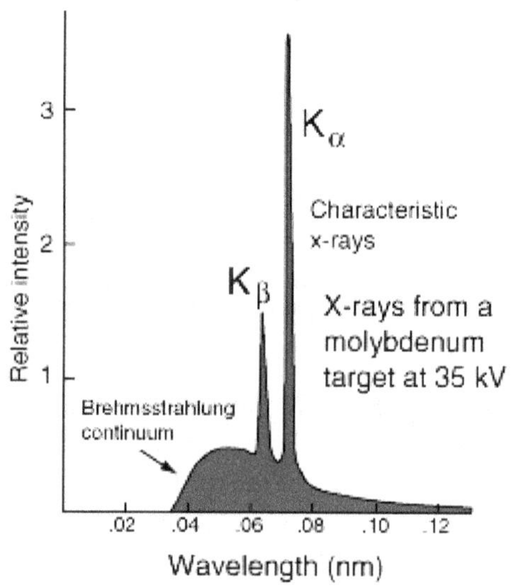

Figure 8.3 Characteristics of X-rays.

X-ray crystallography is a technique used for determining the atomic and molecular structure of a **crystal**, in which the crystalline **atoms** cause a beam of incident **X-rays** to **diffract** into many specific directions. By measuring the angles and intensities of these diffracted beams, a **crystallographer** can produce a three-dimensional picture of the density of **electrons** within the crystal. From this electron density, the mean positions of the atoms in the crystal can be determined, as well as their **chemical bonds**, their **disorder**, and various other information **(Figure 8.4)**.

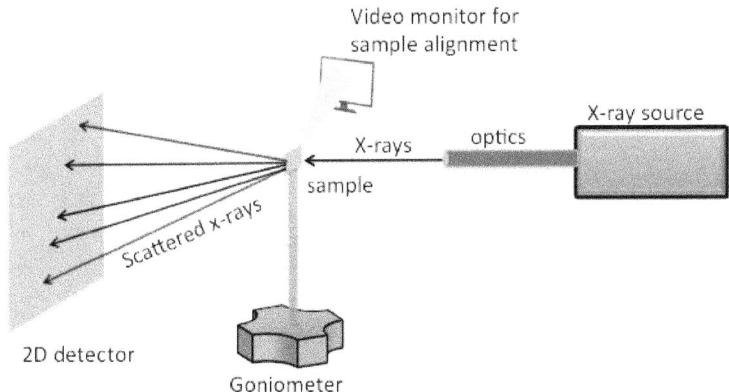

Figure 8.4 Experiment by X-ray crystallography.

In **X-ray diffraction (XRD)** measurement, a **crystal** is mounted on a **goniometer**. The goniometer is used to position the crystal at selected orientations. The crystal is illuminated with a finely focused **monochromatic** beam of X-rays, producing a **diffraction pattern** of regularly spaced spots known as *reflections*. The two-dimensional images taken at different orientations are converted into a three-dimensional model of the density of electrons within the crystal using the mathematical method of **Fourier transforms**, combined with chemical data known for the sample. Poor resolution (fuzziness) or even errors may result if the crystals are too small, or not uniform enough in their internal makeup **(Figure 8.5)**.

Principle of XRD

The diffraction is based on the following

(a) Constructive interference

(b) Distance between two atom or layer (d)

(c) Angle of incident monochromatic X-ray beam

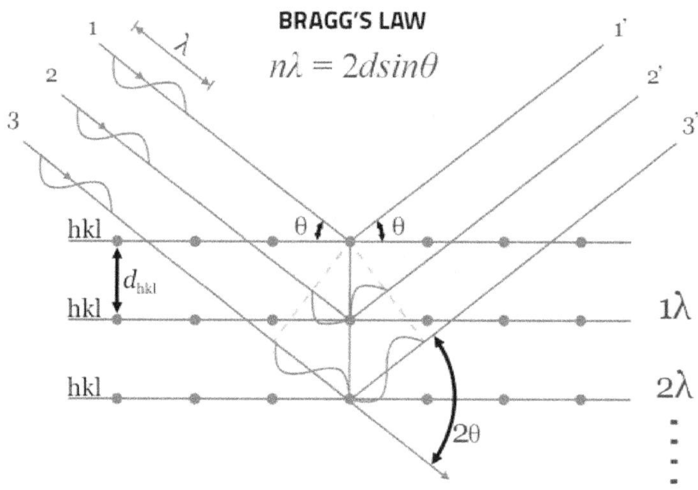

Figure 8.5 Diffraction of X-rays by a crystal.

The XRD pattern is obtained as two theta versus intensity, where x-axis is qualitative scale. An example of Acyclovir XRD pattern, where intensity is directly proportional to crystalline nature (Figure 8.6).

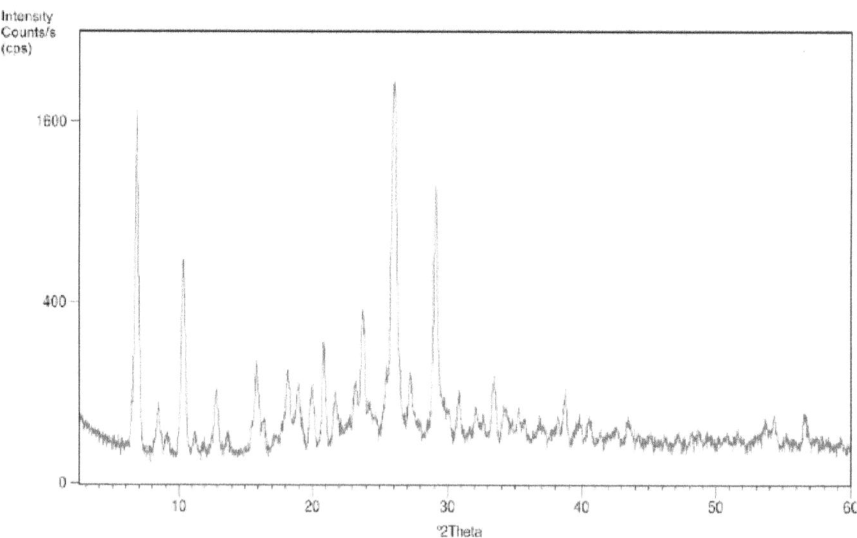

Figure 8.6 XRD pattern of Acyclovir drug.

The below XRD shows (Figure 8.7) the comparative pattern of amorphous form and crystalline form, hence the use information related structure and finger print cannot be identified using amorphous form.

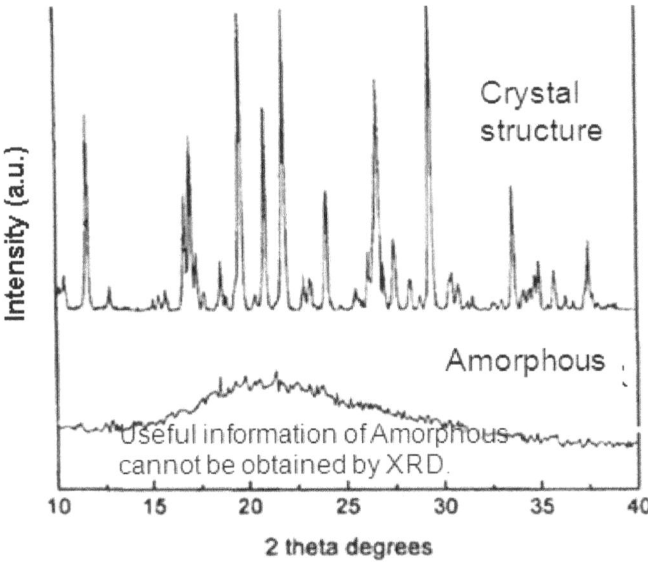

Figure 8.7 XRD pattern of Amorphous and Crystalline forms.

The below XRD (Figure 8.8) is an example of compatibility studies in which XRD pattern of Paracetamol is compared with encapsulated form with PLA and with pure PLA

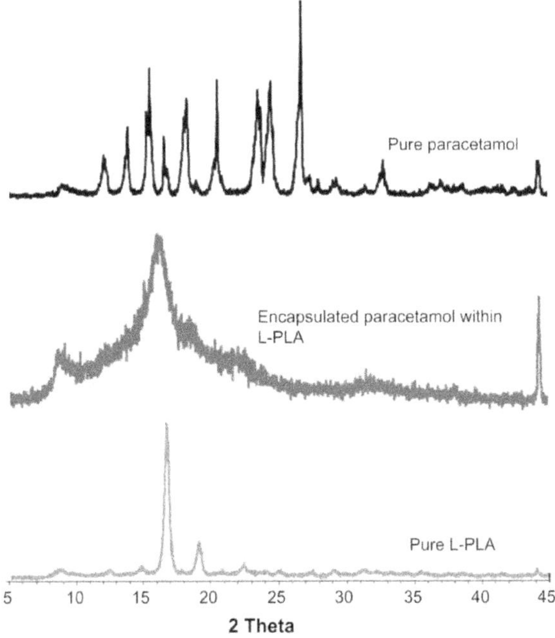

Figure 8.8 XRD pattern of pure Paracetamol compared with encapsulated form with PLA and with pure PLA.

The below is an another example of drug compatibility studies of paracetamol with cholesterol using different formulation technique (Figure 8.9).

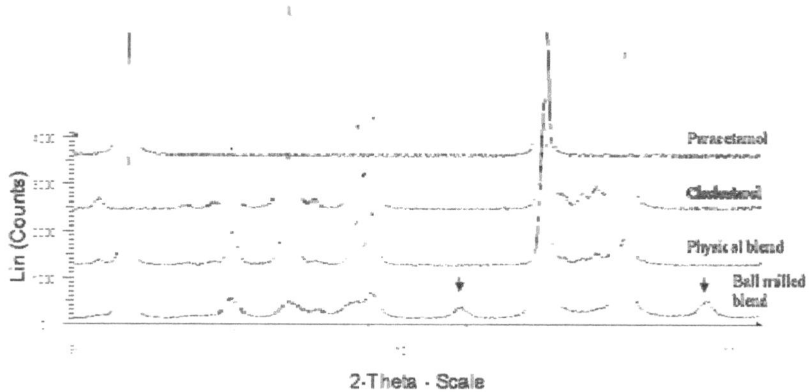

Figure 8.9 XRD pattern of Paracetamol with Cholesterol.

The below shown XRD (Figure 8.10) is example for comparission of Loperamide and its liposomes.

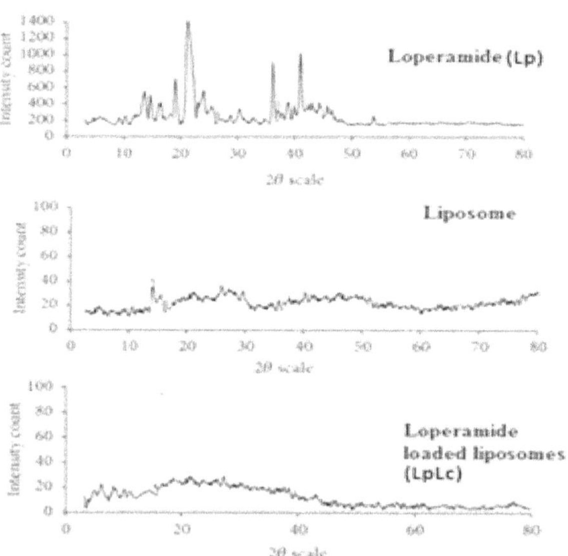

Figure 8.10 XRD pattern for comparison of Loperamide and its liposomes.

Polymorphism Studies

The XRD pattern shown below (Figure 8.11) indicated the different characteristic of peaks (at 2 theta) and intensity for Form I, II, III, IV.

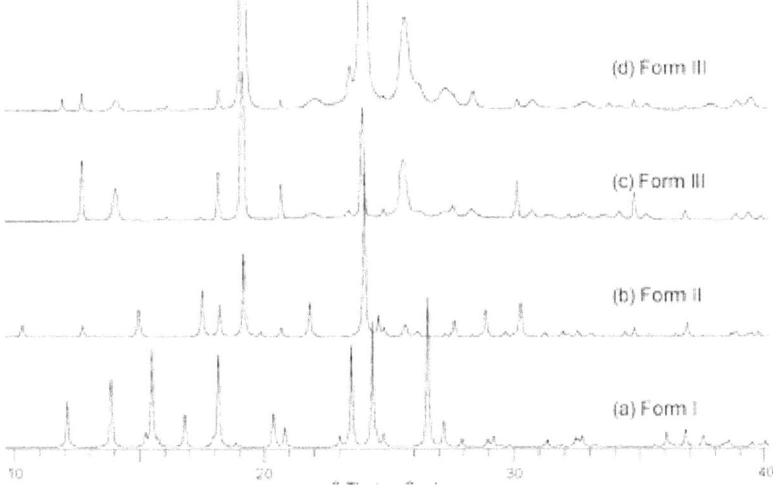

Figure 8.11 XRD pattern for Polymorphism studies.

The following XRD pattern is an example of Control release formulation of Diclofenac in which pure drug (3) is compared with Dosage form (1&2). Where drug shows the more amorphous characteristics. However the intensity pattern around 20 theta scale shows the presence of Diclofenac in the formulation (Figure 8.12).

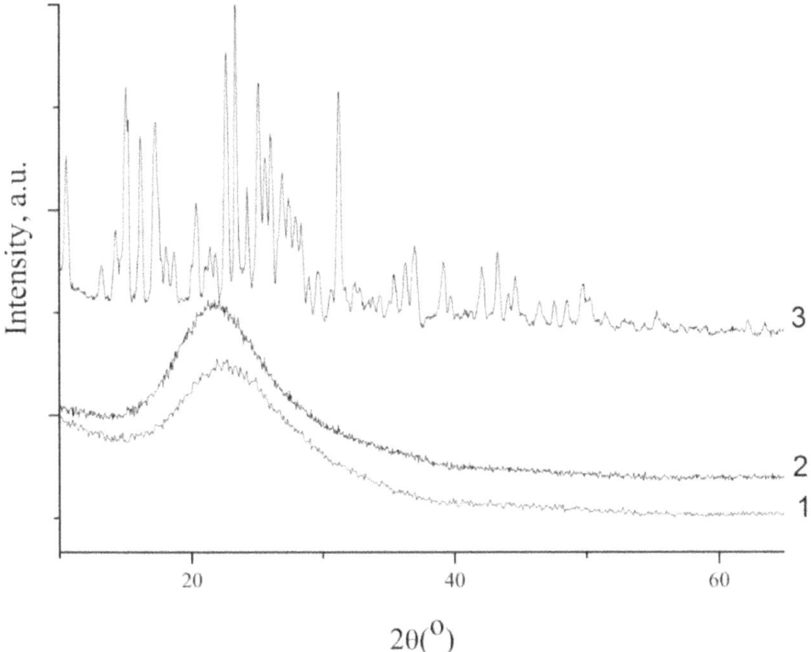

Figure 8.12 XRD pattern of Control release formulation of Diclofenac.

Chapter 9

Scanning Electron Microscopy (SEM)

The **Scanning Electron Microscopy (SEM)** uses a focused beam of high-energy electrons to generate a variety of signals at the surface of solid specimens. The signals that derive from electron-sample interactions reveal the following

- external morphology (texture),
- chemical composition,
- crystalline structure
- Orientation of materials making up the sample.

In most applications, data are collected over a selected area of the surface of the sample, and a 2-dimensional image is generated that displays spatial variations in these properties. Areas ranging from approximately 1 cm to 5 microns in width can be imaged in a scanning mode using conventional SEM techniques (magnification ranging from 20X to approximately 30,000X, spatial resolution of 50 to 100 nm). The SEM is also capable of performing analysis of selected point locations on the sample; this approach is especially useful in qualitatively or semi-quantitatively determining chemical compositions, crystalline structure, and crystal orientations

Scanning Electron microscopy (SEM) Vs Transmission Electron Microscopy (TEM)

SEM detects electrons which are reflected from the **surface** of the sample. TEM detects electrons which went **through** the sample. Thus SEM shows the surface of the sample, and TEM can show its inside (sometimes down to seeing individual atoms, if the TEM is very good and the sample very thin) (Figure 9.1).

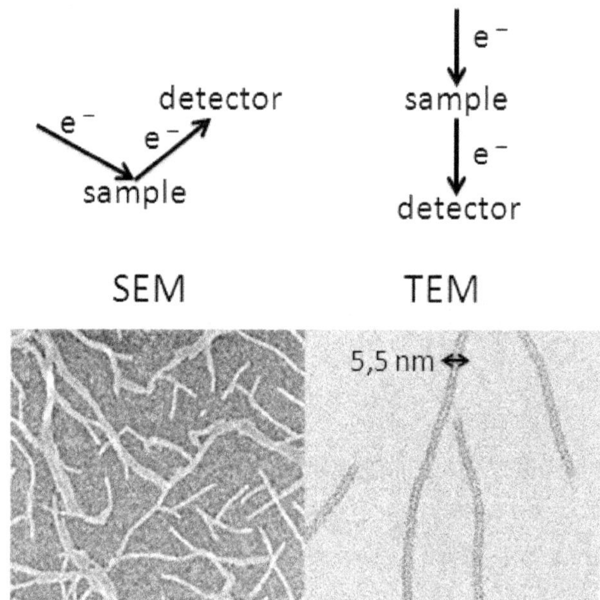

Difference between 2D and 3D Scanning Electron Microscopy

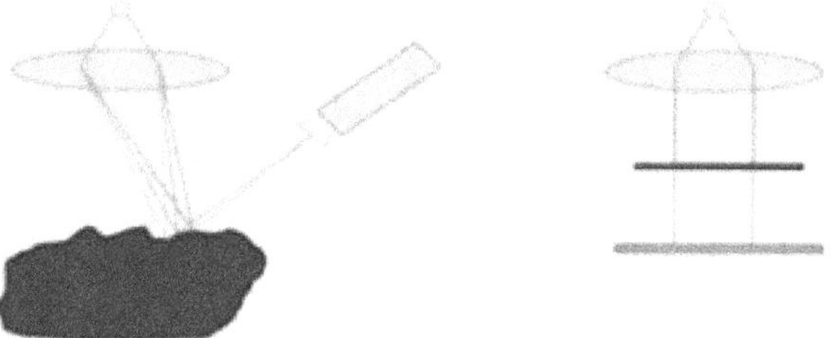

- 3-D
- Beam formation
- Magnification – 2 million
- Resolution – 0.4 nm
- Scans larger areas
- Limitations – conducting samples, charging effect

- 2-D
- Direct imaging
- Magnification – 50 million
- Resolution – 0.5 Å
- Scans thin samples
- Limitations – magnetic samples

Instrumentation of SEM

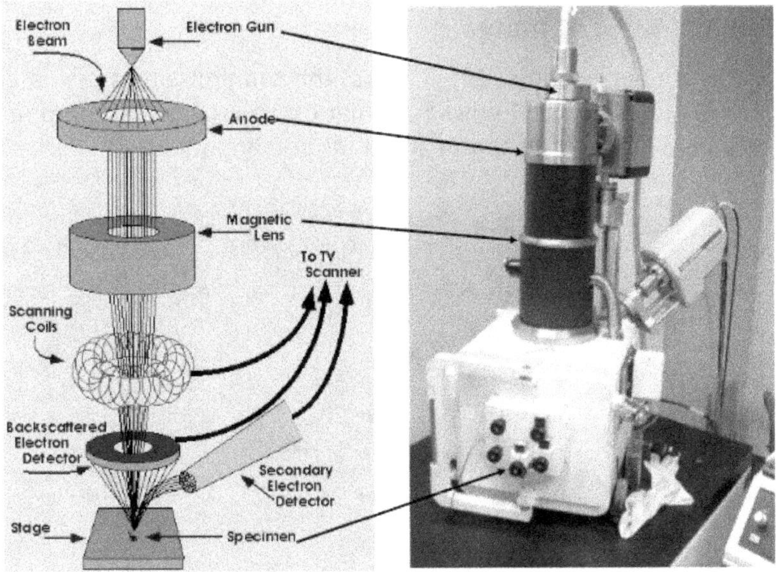

Figure 9.1 Instrumentation of SEM.

Accelerated electrons in an SEM carry significant amounts of kinetic energy, and this energy is dissipated as a variety of signals produced by **electron-sample interactions** when the incident electrons are decelerated in the solid sample. These signals include secondary electrons (that produce SEM images), BackScattered Electrons (**BSE**), diffracted BackScattered Electrons (**DBSE or** EBSD that are used to determine crystal structures and orientations of minerals), photons (**characteristic X-rays** that are used for elemental analysis and continuum X-rays), visible light (**cathode luminescence–CL**), and heat. Secondary electrons and BackScattered of Electrons are commonly used for imaging samples: secondary electrons are most valuable for showing morphology and topography on samples and BackScattered Electrons are most valuable for illustrating contrasts in composition in multiphase samples (i.e. for rapid phase discrimination). **X-ray generation** is produced by inelastic collisions of the incident electrons with electrons in discrete orbitals (shells) of atoms in the sample. As the excited electrons return to lower energy states, they yield X-rays that are of a fixed wavelength (that is related to the difference in energy levels of electrons in different shells for a given element). Thus, characteristic X-rays are produced for each element in a mineral that is "excited" by the electron beam. SEM analysis is considered to be "non-destructive"; that is, x-rays generated by electron interactions do not lead to volume loss of the sample, so it is possible to analyze the same materials repeatedly.

SEM Image Vs TEM Image

The following figure shows (Figure 9.2) the comparison of pollen grain under SEM and TEM. SEM gives information about surface components whereas TEM gives information about inner components.

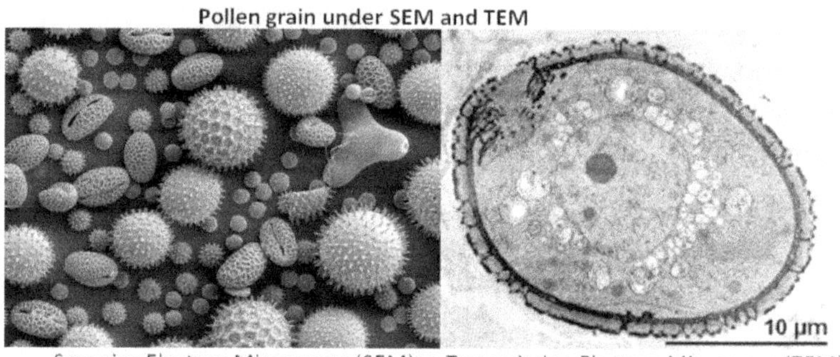

Figure 9.2 Comparison of pollen grain under SEM and TEM.

Pharmaceutical Application of SEM

- Particle size distribution
- De-formulation and Pre-formulation
- Drug load behavior of polymers and lipids
- Crystals studies
- Pharmaceutical assurance on morphological characteristics
- Study of drug release mechanism

Few examples of Pharmaceutical Formulations

1. **Liposomes:** SEM and cross-section TEM images of the oxidized crosslinked P(S-DVB) microspheres before (A and B) and after graft polymerization of AN (C and D) and CMS (F and E), respectively

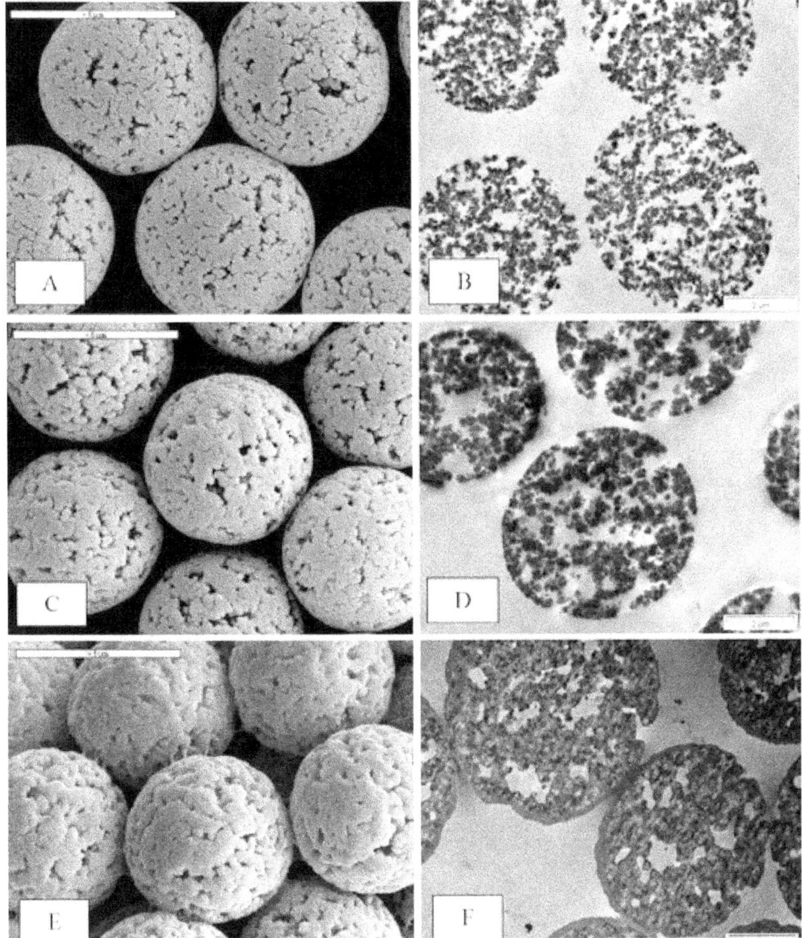

Figure 9.3 SEM and cross-section TEM images of Liposomes.

2. **Microphere:** SEM images of non-porous (A) and porous PLGA microspheres with different particle sizes obtained at stirring speeds of (B) 700 rpm, (C) 800 rpm, (D) 900 rpm (Figure 9.4).

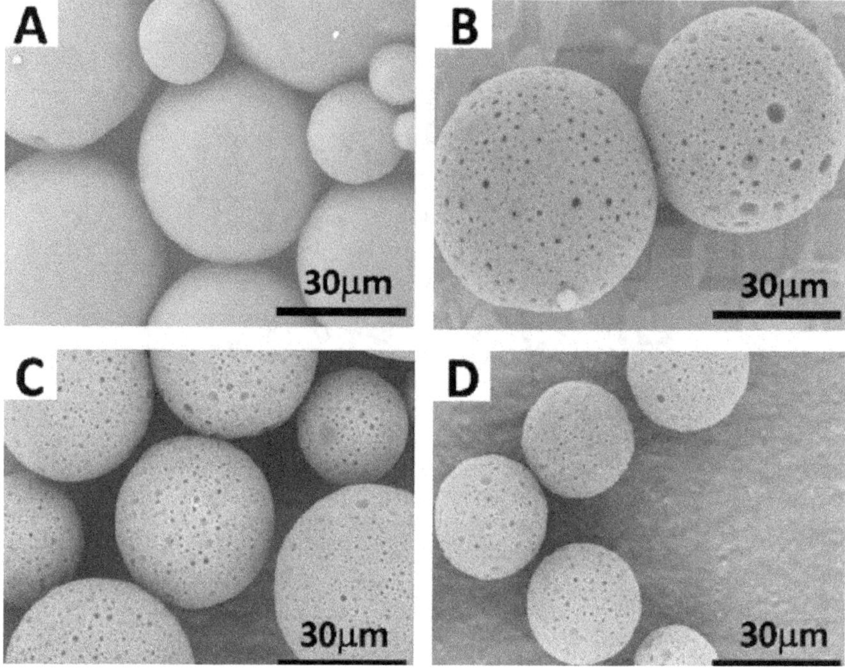

Figure 9.4 SEM images of Microspheres.

Chapter 10

Quantitative Techniques using UV Spectroscopy

UV method can be used for single component and multi-component samples (dosage form)

The method decision can be made based on the following table

Table 10.1 Selection of quantitative method in UV spectroscopy

If standard is not available, but A1%1cm value is known	If Standard available	
	Single component	**Multi-component**
A1%1cm method (IP recommend)	Calibration curve Direct comparison Standard addition	Solvent extraction method Simultaneous analysis Absorbance ratio method Absorption correction Geometric correction Orthogonal polynomial Derivative spectrometry H-Point addition method Least square approximation method

Single Component Analysis

Direct Analysis: Essentially all compounds containing conjugated double bond or aromatic rings, and many inorganic species absorb light in the UV-visible regions. In these techniques the substance to be determined is dissolved in suitable solvent and diluted to the required concentration by appropriate dilutions and absorbance is measured.

Indirect Analysis: (Analysis after addition of some reagent) indirect methods are based on the conversion of the analyte by a chemical reagent that has different spectral properties. Chemical derivatization may be adopted for any of the several reasons. 1) If the analyte absorbs weakly in the UV region. 2) The interference from irrelevant absorption may be avoided by converting the analyte to a derivative, which absorbs in the visible region, where irrelevant absorption is negligible. 3) This technique can be used to improve the selectivity of the assay in presence of other UV radiation absorbing substance. 4) Cost.

1. **$A^{1\%}_{1cm}$ method:** There are two form of Beers-Lambert law, which can be used for quantification purpose

Based on molar absorbance	Based on Specific absorbance
$A = \epsilon \times b \times C$	$A = A^{1\%}_{1cm} \times b \times C$
C – measure as moles per liter	C – measured as g /100 ml
• Molar absorbance defined as an absorbance of 1 molar solution at specific wavelength. • Molar extinction co-efficient or molar aborptivity are used to assess the UV absorption	• Specific absorbance defined as an absorbance of 1 g /100 ml solutions at specific wavelength • It is recommended by IP 2014 • More suitable for quantification when standards are not available.

Both values can be converted to each other by using the following formula,

$$A^{1\%}_{1cm} = (10 \times \epsilon) / \text{Molecular weight}$$

Unless otherwise prescribed, measure the absorbance at the prescribed wavelength using a path length of 1 cm and at 20 ± 1 °C. Unless otherwise prescribed, the measurements are carried out with reference to the same solvent or the same mixture of solvents. The absorbance of the solvent measured against air and at the prescribed wavelength shall not exceed 0.4 and is preferably less than 0.2. Plot the absorption spectrum with absorbance or function of absorbance as ordinate against wavelength or function of wavelength as abscissa. Where a monograph gives a single value for the position of an absorption maximum, it is understood that the value obtained may differ by not more than ± 2 nm.

2. **Calibration curve technique: Regression method**: Prepare a series of standard concentrations (S1, S2, S3, S4, S5) and read absorbance and establish linearity by taking concentration in X axis and milli absorbance or absorbance in Y axis. Validate that the regression coefficient is more than 0.99. then use the equation for calculating the unknown sample (Figure 10.1).

$$Y = mx \pm c$$

$$X = (Y \pm C)/m$$

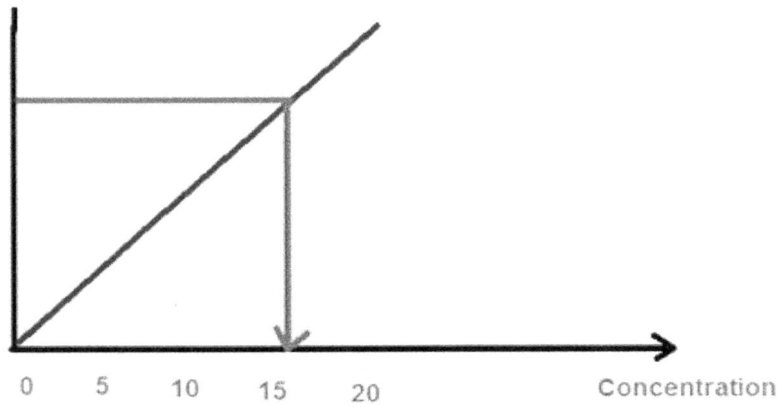

Figure 10.1 Linear regression by UV Spectroscopic technique (Beer's Law).

Interpolation method: If the intercept C = 0 (when x = 0, y = 0), the interpolation method can be used (Figure 10.2).

Figure 10.2 Interpolation of Calibration curve for Unknown sample.

3. **Direct comparison method:** Standard (S) and Test (t) have to be prepared to parallel concentrations and the respective absorbances have to be noted (As, At).

$$As = Cs, \text{ where } At = Ct$$

Hence $At/As = Ct/Cs$

Based on the above equation the unknown concentration can be determined. But replicate analysis is essential.

4. **Standard Addition technique:** The method of **standard addition** is a type of quantitative analysis approach often used in **analytical chemistry** whereby the standard is added directly to the aliquots of analyzed sample. This method is used in situations where sample matrix also contributes to the analytical signal, a situation known as the **matrix effect**, thus making it impossible to compare the analytical signal between sample and standard using the traditional **calibration curve** approach (Figure 10.3).

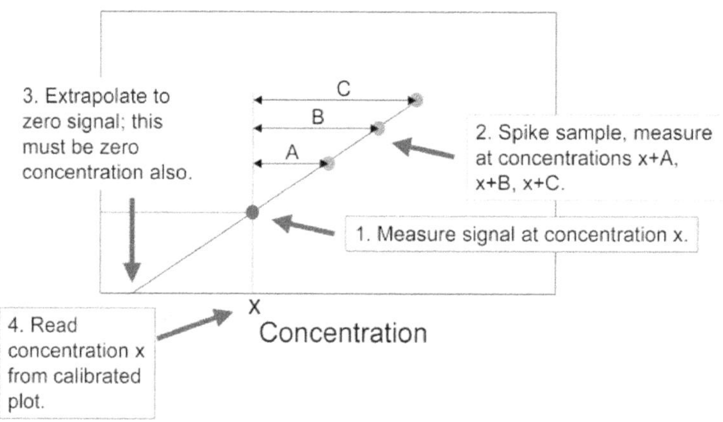

Figure 10.3 Standard addition technique - Quantitative analysis approaches.

Multi-Component Analysis by UV Spectroscopy

The most suitable method s in Pharmaceutical analysis are explained in this section

Simultaneous Equation Method (Vierdot's Method)

If a sample contains two absorbing drugs (x and y) each of which absorbs at the λ max of the other , it may be possible to determine both drugs by the technique of simultaneous equation (vierodt's method) provided that certain criteria apply.

The information required is:

- The absorptivities of x at λ_1 and λ_2, a_{x1} and a_{x2} respectively
- The absorptivities of y at λ_1 and λ_2, a_{y1} and a_{y2} respectively
- The absorbance of the diluted sample at λ_1 and λ_2, a_1 and a_2 respectively.

Conditions to Apply

Criteria for obtaining maximum precision have been suggested by Glenn. According to him absorbance ratio place limits on the relative concentrations of the components of the mixture.

$$(A_2/A_1) / (a_{x2}/a_{x1}) \text{ and } (a_{y2}/a_{y1}) / (A2/A1)$$

- The criteria are that the ratios should lie outside the range 0.1-2.0 for the precise determination of y and x respectively.

- These criteria are satisfied only when the λmax of the two components are reasonably dissimilar.

- An additional criterion is that the two components do not interact chemically, thereby negating the initial assumption that the total absorbance is the sum of the individual absorbance (Figure 10.4).

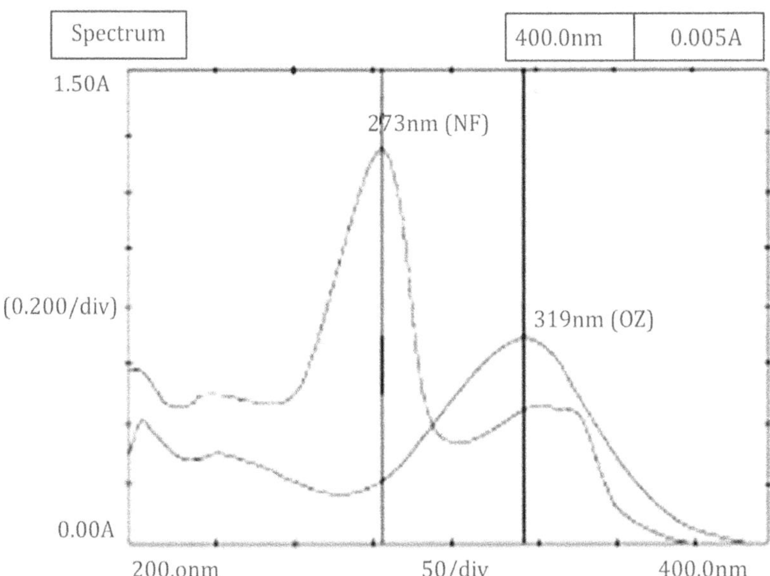

For example Drug X (λ_1: 273 nm), Drug Y (λ_1: 319 nm)

Figure 10.4 UV spectra of drug X and Y.

If Cx and Cy be the concentration of x and y respectively in the diluted samples, then

$$@ \lambda_1: \quad A_1 = a_{x1}bc_x + a_{y1}bc_y \qquad \text{............ (1)}$$

$$@\lambda_2: \quad A_2 = a_{x2}bc_x + a_{y2}bc_y \qquad \text{......... (2)}$$

Rearrange Equation (2)

C_y = $(A_2 - a_{x2} c_x)$ / ay2

Substituting for c_y in eq. (1) and rearranging gives

C_x = $(A_2 a_{y1} - A_1 a_{y2})$ / $(ax_2 a_{y1} - a_{x1} a_{y2})$

C_y = $(A_1 a_{x2} - A_2 a_{x1})$ / $(ax_2 a_{y1} - a_{x1} a_{y2})$

✓ $\lambda2$= λmax of drug 2

✓ Cx = concentration of drug 1 in mixture

✓ Cy = concentration of drug 2 in mixture

✓ ax1= absorptivity of drug 1 at $\lambda1$

✓ ax2= absorptivity of drug 1 at $\lambda2$

✓ ay1= absorptivity of drug 2 at $\lambda1$

✓ ay2 = absorptivity of drug 2 at $\lambda2$

✓ A1 = absorbance of mixture at $\lambda1$

✓ A2 = absorbance of mixture at $\lambda2$

Absorbance Ratio Method (Q - Analysis)

The Absorbance ratio method is a method for simultaneous estimation of two components depending upon the property that the ratio of absorbances at any two wavelengths is a constant value independent of concentration or pathlength. Absorption ratio method is used for the ratio of the absorption at two selected wavelength one of which is the iso-absorptive point and other being the λmax of one of the two components. In absorbance ratio method (Q-analysis), the primary requirement for developing a method for analysis is that the entire spectra should follow the Beer's law at all the wavelength, which was fulfilled in case of both these drugs.

Example: Norfloxacin (NF: X drug) and Ornidazole (OZ: Y drug), 297 nm is the isosbestic point considered to be $\lambda1$, 318 nm shall be considered as $\lambda2$ (Figure 10.5).

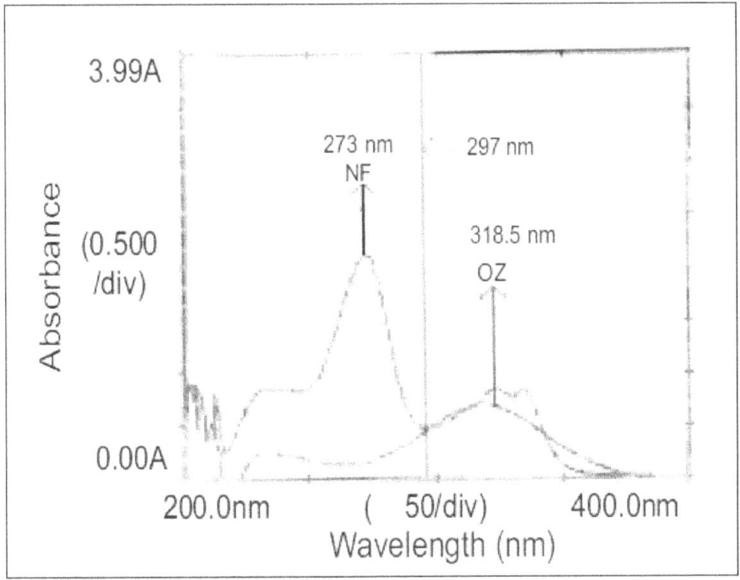

Figure 10.5 UV spectra of Norfloxacin and Ornidazole.

Calculations

Drug name	$\lambda 1$ (iso) 264nm	$\lambda 2$ 249 nm
Drug 1 (X) - PCM	$A/Cx = ax_1$ $A/Cy = ay_1$ @ Isobestic Point $ax1 = ay1$	$A/Cx = ax_2$
Drug 2 (Y) -PP		$A/Cy = ay_2$
Mixture (X+Y)	A1	A2

If,

Qx	Qy	QM
ax2/ax1	ay2/ay1	A2/A1

If 264 nm ($\lambda 1$) is isosbestic point, if 249 nm is $\lambda 2$

$$Cx = \frac{Q_m - Q_y}{Q_x - Q_y} \times \frac{A_1}{ax_1}$$

$$Cy = \frac{Q_m - Q_x}{Q_y - Q_x} \times \frac{A_1}{ay_1}$$

$$Q_m = \frac{\text{Absorbance of sample solution at 249 nm (A2)}}{\text{Absorbance of sample solution at 264 nm (A1)}}$$

$$Q_x = \frac{\text{Absorptivity of PCM at 249 nm}}{\text{Absorptivity of PCM at 264 nm}}$$

$$Q_y = \frac{\text{Absorptivity of PP at 249 nm}}{\text{Absorptivity of PP at 264 nm}}$$

Derivative Spectroscopy

Derivative spectroscopy involves the conversion of a normal spectra to its first, second or higher derivative spectra. The normal spectrum is known as fundamental, zero order or D0 spectra. The first derivative spectrum (D1) is a plot of the rate of change of absorbance with wavelength against wavelength, i.e. plot of $\Delta A/\Delta \lambda$ vs. λ. The second derivative spectrum is a plot of $\Delta 2\ A/\ \Delta \lambda 2$ vs. λ. Not only can the first and second derivative of the absorbance spectrum be obtained, but up to the fourth derivative is possible. However, as the differentiation order increases, the noise increases as well, and if a lower derivative is fine, going to higher derivatives is a waste of time and effort. The next slide will show how mathematically the derivatives are graphed.

To find the quantitative estimation of binary mixtures using the derivative spectroscopy, we first need to find out the Zero Crossing Points (ZCP) for both the components (A and B). After that we must select the ZCP for A and B so that particular ZCP of other component show as remarkable absorbance. Then, we must prepare the calibration curve of A at the ZCP of B and of B at the ZCP of A. In doing this we can find out the unknown concentration using this calibration curves.

In simultaneous analysis, ZCP is taken for drug quantification. Example 263 nm is suitable for quantification of dark line spectra of compounds; whereas 348 nm is suitable for dotted line compounds (Figure 10.6).

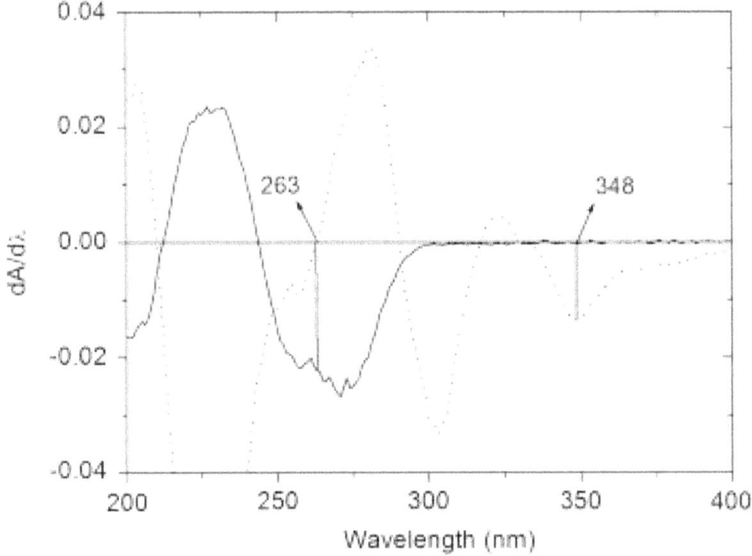

Figure 10.6 Quantitative estimation of binary mixtures by Derivative spectroscopy.

Then absorbance are measured as usual as that of calibration curve method. Below is the overlay spectra of series of standard for one drug (Figure 10.7).

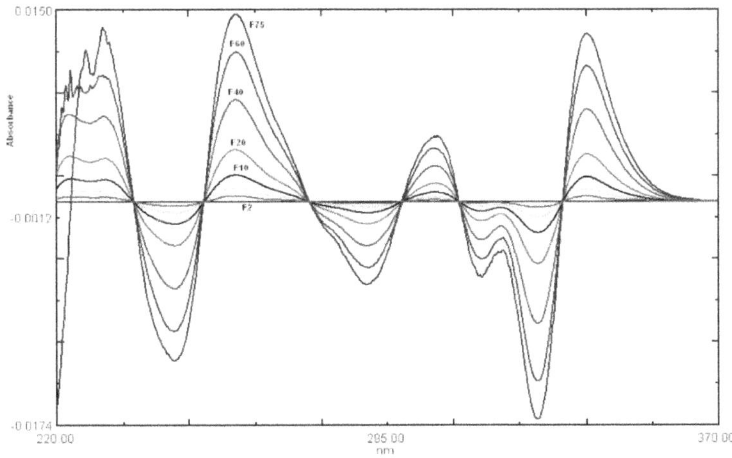

Figure 10.7 Overlay UV- Derivative spectra of series of standard for one drug.

For other methods, please refer the reported research article for better understanding.

Quantitative Application of IR Spectroscopy

It is also called quantitative IR spectroscopy. It can be used for the following

1. Simple Analysis for liquids and Solids
2. Multi-component analysis

Analysis of Liquid: The quantitative analysis of a component in solution can be successfully carried only if suitable band in the spectrum of the component of interest. The band which we choose should be

- with high molar absorptivity
- Should not overlap with other bands
- Free from other interference and solvents bands
- Should be symmetrical, and
- Should prove linearity for absorbance versus concentration.

NOTE: Most simple quantitative infrared methods uses the intensities of the C=O, N–H or O–H groups. Among all C=O stretching band is the most commonly used because it is the most intense symmetrical than other functional. And also C=O is not as susceptible as the O–H and N–H bands to chemical change or hydrogen bonding.

Analysis of Solids (Baseline technique): These are more susceptible to errors because of

- The scattering of radiation
- Difficulty in measuring the pathlength.

However, above error can be overcome with the use of "Mull" an internal standard is used. The calibration plot is drawn between ratio of the absorbance of the analyte to that of the internal standard Vs concentration of the analyte. It is must that standards and samples should be analysed under same conditions.

NOTE: The standard must possess the following:
- have a simple spectrum with very few bands;
- be stable to heat and not absorb moisture;
- be easily reduced to a particle size less than the incident radiation without lattice deformation;
- be non-toxic, giving clear discs in a short time;
- be readily available in the pure state.
- Some common standards used include calcium carbonate, sodium azide, napthalene and lead thiocyanate.

The following figure shows (Figure 10.8) the calculation of absorbance for the selected band in series of concentrations and sample. Po, PT is measured from the baseline, in modern instruments; baseline correction is done automatically to 98-100%. Most of the quantitative IR spectrums are obtained in absorption mode.

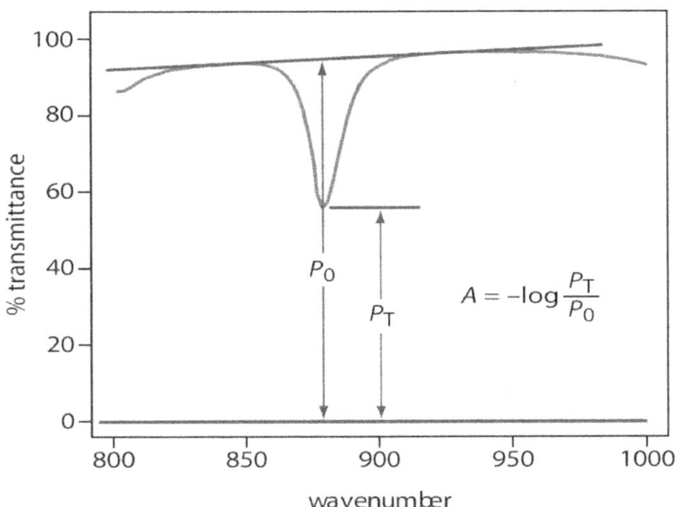

Figure 10.8 Quantitative analysis by IR spectrum (Baseline technique).

The below presented IR spectrum an (Figure 10.9) example of absorption mode, where series of concentrations shown increase in absorption at 1741 cm^{-1} for C=O. Remaining bands are low resolution and less intense than carbonyl group.

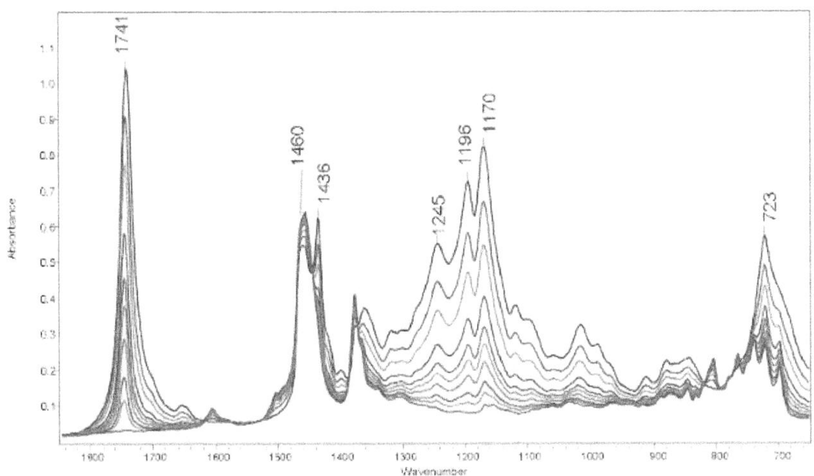

Figure 10.9 IR spectrum showing increase in absorption at 1741 cm-1 for C=O.

Multi-component analysis: It is less common in Pharmaceutical analysis because low selectivity and less Precise and Accuracy.

Quantitative analysis by ATR: The use of attenuated total reflection (ATR) accessories in conjunction with Fourier Transform Infrared (FTIR) spectrometers is now commonplace. This accessory provides for the non-destructive measurement of samples with little or no preparation. Most samples can be directly applied to the Internal Reflection Element (IRE) of an ATR without time-consuming dilution with matrices such as Nujol or KBr. The ATR accessory also allows for easy analysis of liquid samples with just a single drop required, applied directly to the IRE crystal. However, by the nature of their design, ATR accessories absorb infrared radiation and consequently reduce the amount of energy that reaches the infrared detector. The attenuation caused by these accessories typically varies from 70–90%.

Chapter 11

LC-NMR and Q-NMR

LC-NMR

Analytical methods that connect chromatographs and spectrometers online are called hyphenated techniques. LC-NMR combines 2 techniques-Liquid chromatography (LC) and Nuclear magnetic resonance (NMR). It involves a HPLC separation followed by the detection of separated components by UV or other methods & ultimately NMR analysis. The on-line coupling of high-performance liquid chromatography (HPLC principles to high-resolution NMR spectrometers offers a powerful tool for analyzing and characterizing complex chemical mixtures without the need of chemical separation. LC-NMR promises to be of great value in the analysis of complex mixtures of all types, particularly the analysis of natural products and drug-related metabolites in bio-fluids, unknown components like impurities and synthetic polymers. The LC-NMR Instrument is shown below (Figure 11.1).

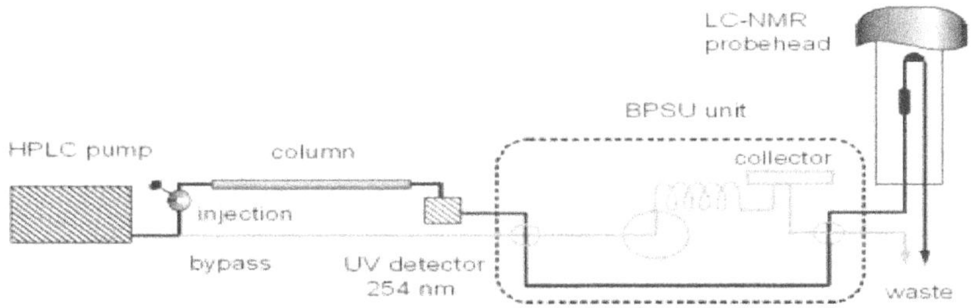

Figure 11.1 LC-NMR Instrumentation.

An example of different types such

- on flow
- Stop-flow
- Loop Transfer
- SPE elution

Are shown in following modern instrument of LC-NMR (Figure 11.2).

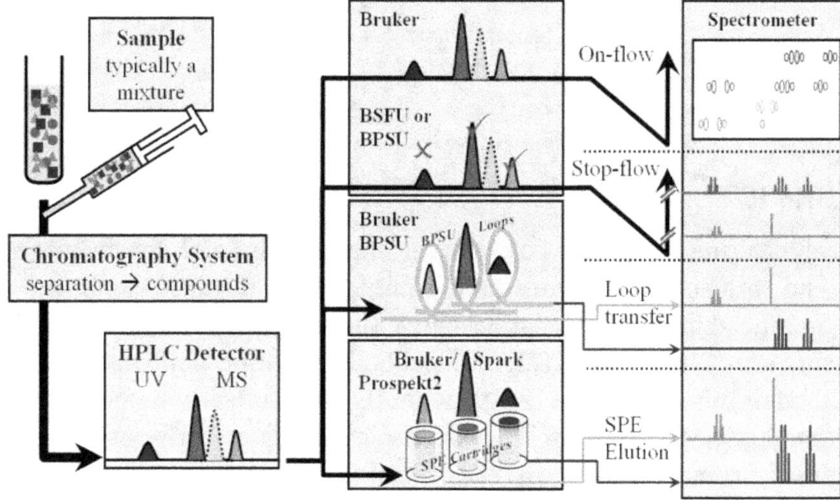

Figure 11.2 Instrument of LC-NMR.

Modes of LC-NMR

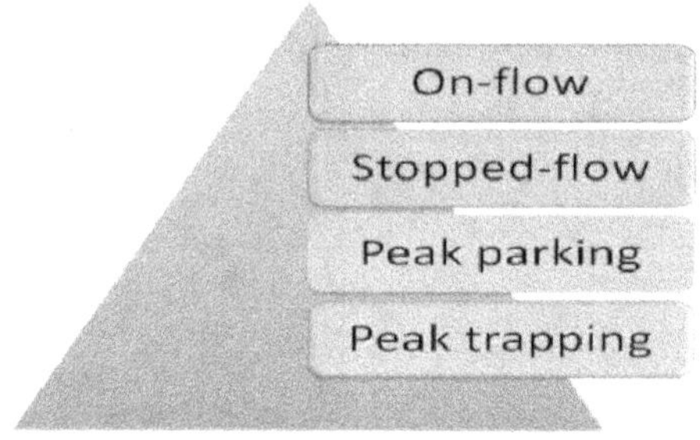

Technology to improve LC-NMR Sensitivity

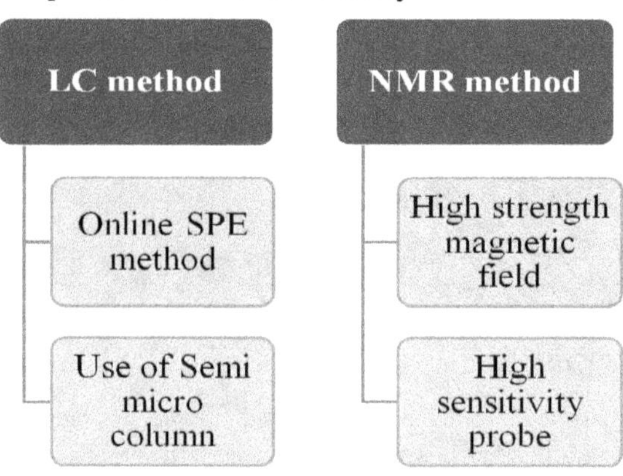

Other than this, solvent suppression methods like pre-saturation and wet methods also used. (Advantage and disadvantage of LC-NMR. An example of LC-NMR spectrum is shown below (Figure 11.3).)

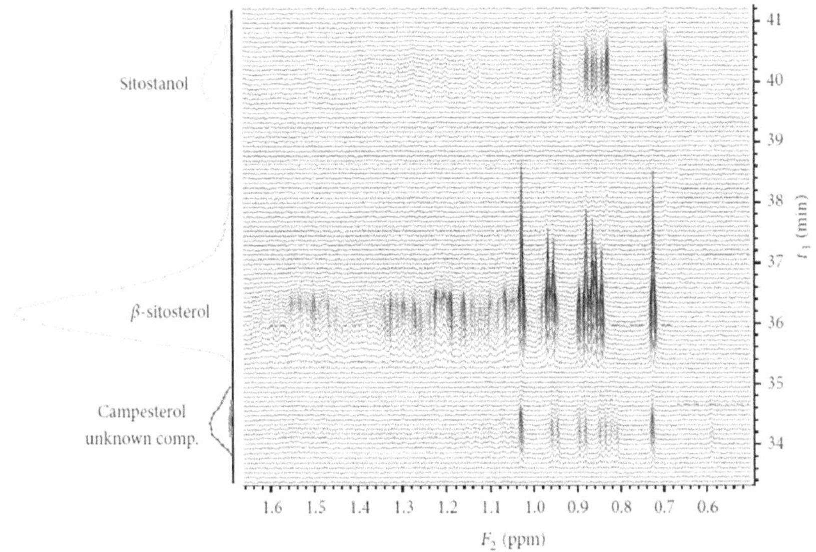

Figure 11.3 LC NMR Spectra (Mixed view).

Advantages of LC NMR

- The information between the 2 techniques is so orthogonal. HPLC resolve "complexity of a mixture" by separation whereas NMR resolves any structure question.
- The NMR can determine if the LC peak impure.
- It is non-destructive technique
- Sample can be stored for analysis by another method.

Disadvantages of LC NMR

- High cost
- Frequently stopping the pump affects the resolution.
- Operator training requirements
- Doing LC-NMR MS requires a unique set of skills.
- Difficulty in solvent selection
- Flow systems can clog up, and get dirty and be hard to clean.

Application of LC-NMR

1. Separation and characterization of peptide libraries.

2. Combinatorial chemistry, phytochemical analysis, drug discovery.

3. Identification of drug impurities.

4. Characterization of isomers of acid glucoronides and vitamin A derivatives.

5. Characterization of endogeneous and xenobiotics metabolites directly from Biological fluid

6. Combination of LC-NMR and LC-MS.

7. Polymer analysis.

8. LC-NMR allowed the differentiation of isomers and identification without reference compounds.

9. Drug metabolism (to analyze biofluids [I.e., urine or plasma]).

High-Performance LC-NMR

This is achieved by two technologies

1. **Technique for increasing sensitivity on the chromatography:** This is by the use of column internal diameter about 2 mm (semi-micro columns). This is called peak concentration method best suited for LC-NMR. The peak concentration is achieved by reduction of column volume using semi-micro column (1/5 of a conventional column). Furthermore the flow rate also reduced to of 0.2 mL/min, hence, the peak width for 120 μL flow-cell expands to around 40 seconds is possible to reduced to 8 seconds (Figure 11.4). In addition, pretreatment methods such as preparative HPLC and solid phase extraction (SPE) etc., need to be implemented. The online SPE method is most commonly used in LC-NMR as a technique to concentrate trace components.

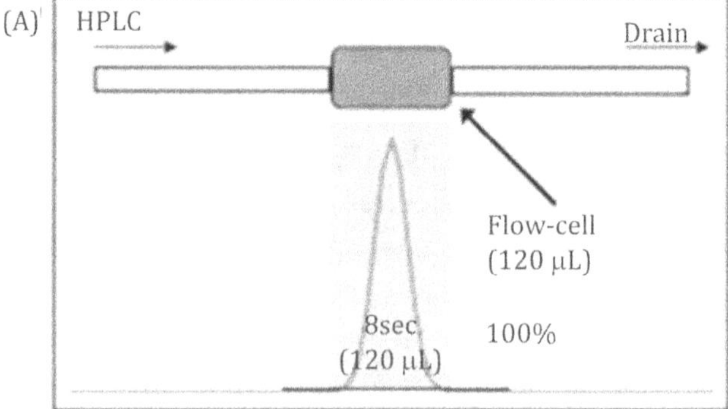

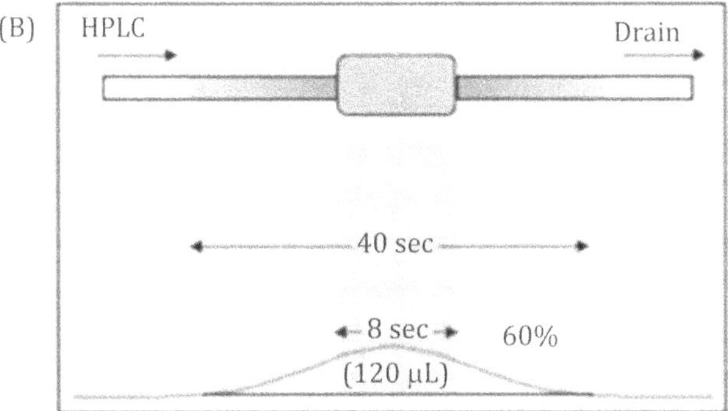

Figure 11.4 Peak concentration in LC-NMR.

2. **Technique for increasing sensitivity on the NMR equipment:** In general, both highly magnetic field magnets and high-sensitivity probes can be used in the achievement of high-performance LC-NMR. Usually the NMR detection sensitivity is proportional to the magnetic field strength (to the 3/2 power). The stronger the external magnetic field always yields the better sensitivity. So, the magnetic field strength has reached 800 MHz or more can be better suited for LC-NMR (Figure 11.5).

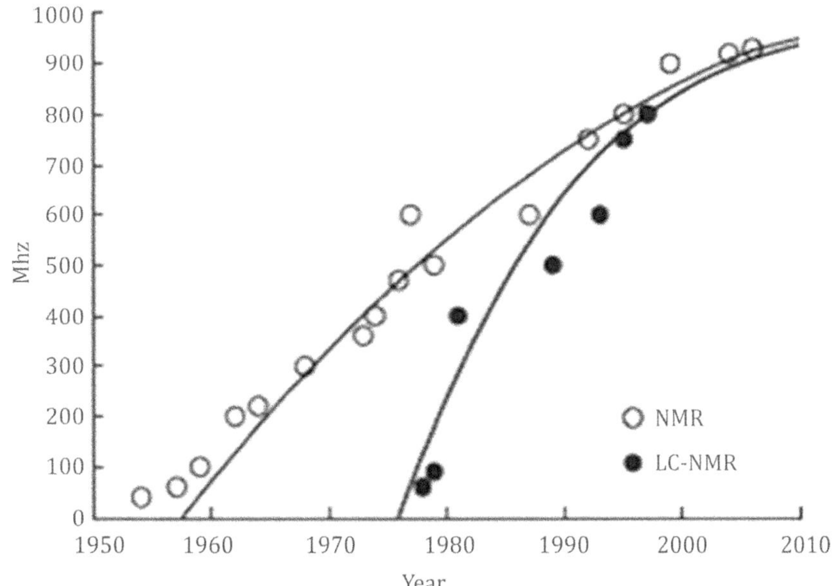

Figure 11.5(a) Sensitivity and magnetic field in NMR and LC-NMR.

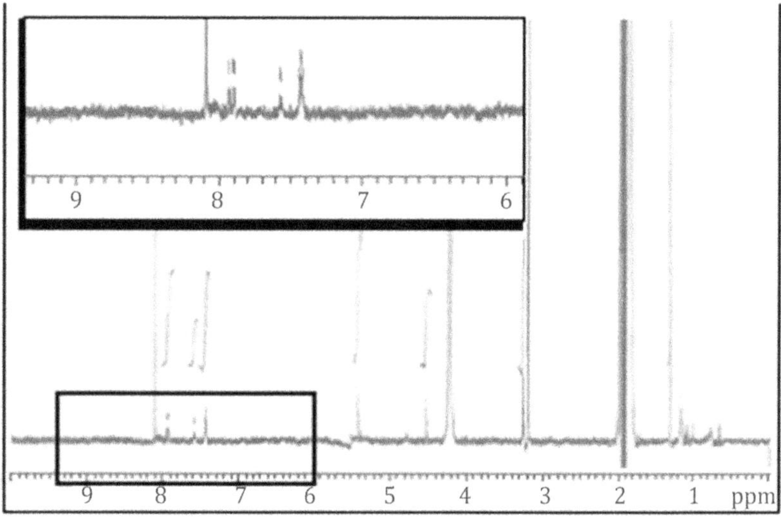

Figure 11.5(b) LC-NMR Spectra at 800 MHZ.

3. **Technique for solvent suppression:** In the beginning of LC-NMR, due to disturbed the measurements by proton signals, LC-NMR was limited to low polarity compound which employed carbon tetrachloride, tetrachloroethylene and Freon as solvents (mobile phase). Once the reversed phase mode has introduced in LCNMR with ODS columns, usually there is overalp of aromatic compounds signals with signals from mobile phase solvents, residual water in deuterium oxide, acetonitrile and methanol. The combined methods of both selective excitation pulses and a pulsed field gradient (PFG) could be used to suppress multiple solvent peaks effects. This is a solvent elimination technique currently used with LC-NMR.

4. **Loop Storage method:** This is the method used in simultaneous analysis of multiple components. In this method multi-components were separated by column and fractionated in sample loops. Later, samples are transferred from loop to the flow-cell in order and were measured.

Quantification Technique (Q-NMR)

While used most often for structural analysis, NMR is increasingly being considered as a critical quantitative tool. NMR is most powerful when used quantitatively, as the integrated intensity of a resonance signal is directly proportional to the number of nuclei represented by that signal. In addition, all protons across the spectrum are equally sensitive, so determination of quantitative results does not require the need for compound-specific extinction coefficients or calibrations. NMR has been used to determine concentrations of synthetic and biosynthetic products, fine chemicals, and pharmaceuticals, as well as metabolites, catabolites, and endogenous compounds in biological fluids1. Quantitative NMR (QNMR) has been shown to be particularly useful in metabolomics, drug discovery and analysis, and natural product analysis.

Quantitative NMR possesses the required accuracy and precision to become a routine quantitative tool in many analytical laboratories. Chemical referencing with internal standards can provide accurate quantification, but this technique is tedious and contaminates the sample. Several electronic referencing approaches have also been used in an attempt to provide accurate and precise quantitative results, such as ERETIC (Electronic Referencing to access in vivo Concentrations), PIG (Pulse Into Gradient), ARTSI (Amplitude-corrected Referencing Through Signal Injection) and QUANTAS (Quantification by Artificial Signal). However, these methods are limited in scope and/or inherently error-prone 3-7. Accurate and precise qNMR of small molecule organic compounds can be attained easily using only absolute integration of an external concentration standard and 1D spectra, given an NMR platform that is highly stable and linear.

Selection of Internal Standards for Q-NMR

With NMR, pure standard compound (which can be structurally unrelated to our analyte) that contains the nucleus of interest and has a resonance that does not overlap those of our analyte. The analyte concentration can then be determined relative to this standard compound. The requirement for lack of overlap means that most standards have simple NMR spectra, often producing only singlet resonances. Additional requirements for standards to be used for quantitative analysis are that they:

- are chemically inert
- have low volatility
- have similar solubility characteristics as the analyte
- have reasonable T1 relaxation times

Examples: TMS, Dioxane, Dimethyl furan, Potassium hydrogen Phthalate, Trimethyl silyl d4 propionic acids. TMS and dioxane are chemical shift reference compounds commonly used in organic solvents. However they do not make good quantitation standards because they suffer from high volatility.

Based on Integration

Analyte Concentration = (Normalized Area "X" / Normalized Area IS) ×
Standard Concentration

Example: The quantification of X using TSP as internal standard is
shown in below figure

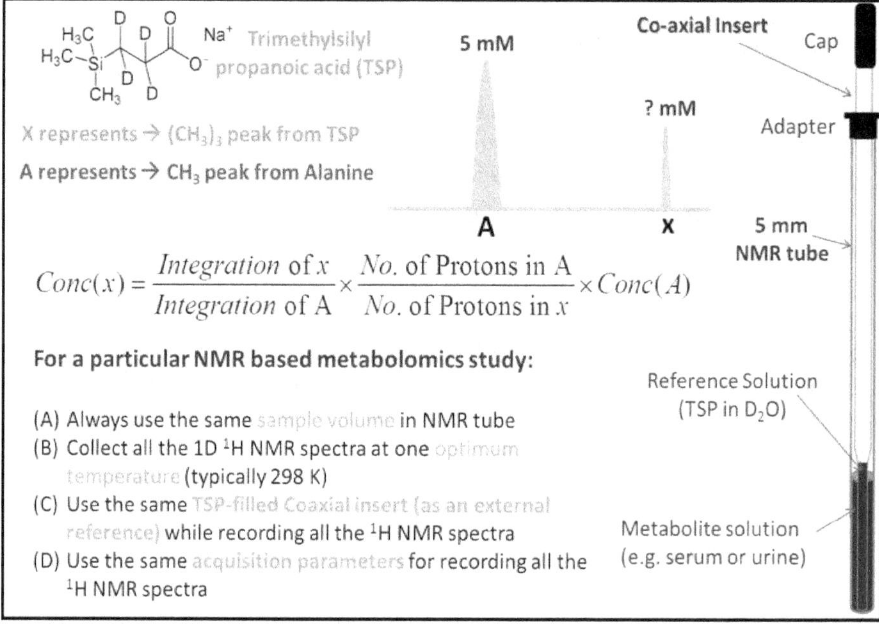

$$Conc(x) = \frac{Integration\ of\ x}{Integration\ of\ A} \times \frac{No.\ of\ Protons\ in\ A}{No.\ of\ Protons\ in\ x} \times Conc(A)$$

Based on NMR Signals Relative Units

The quantification can also be done based on relative units Vs
concentration. Below figure (Figure 11.6) is the example of calibration
curve for quantification of total lipids using 1D NMR.

New Development in LC-NMR

1. LC-SPE-NMR/MS

2. 2D-NMR (HMBC and HSQC)

3. LC-CD-NMR

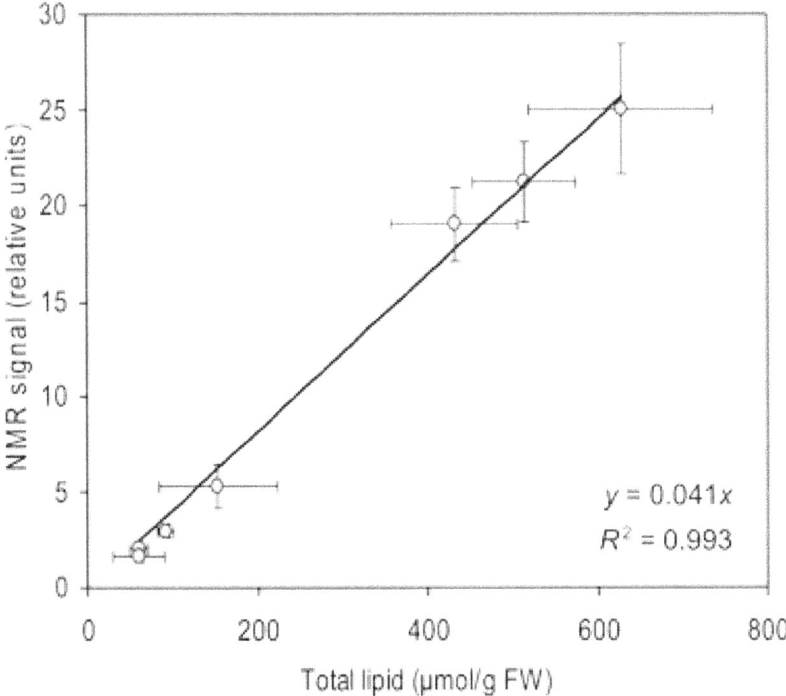

Figure 11.6 Calibration curve for quantification of total lipids using 1D NMR.

Integrated LC-MS and LC-NMR techniques in structure determination. LC-NMR and LC-MS can be inveterately used for structure identification especially in impurity profiling. This added the advantage of structure elucidation with isolation procedure. The schematic chart is shown below,

Chiral LC-CD-NMR, can simultaneously analyze both stereo-isomers and impurities without the use of analytical standards. The trace amount of optical isomers that are included in bulk drugs (technical materials) as byproducts and impurities are identified from CD (Circular dichorism) spectra and NMR spectra, and their elution positions are identified.

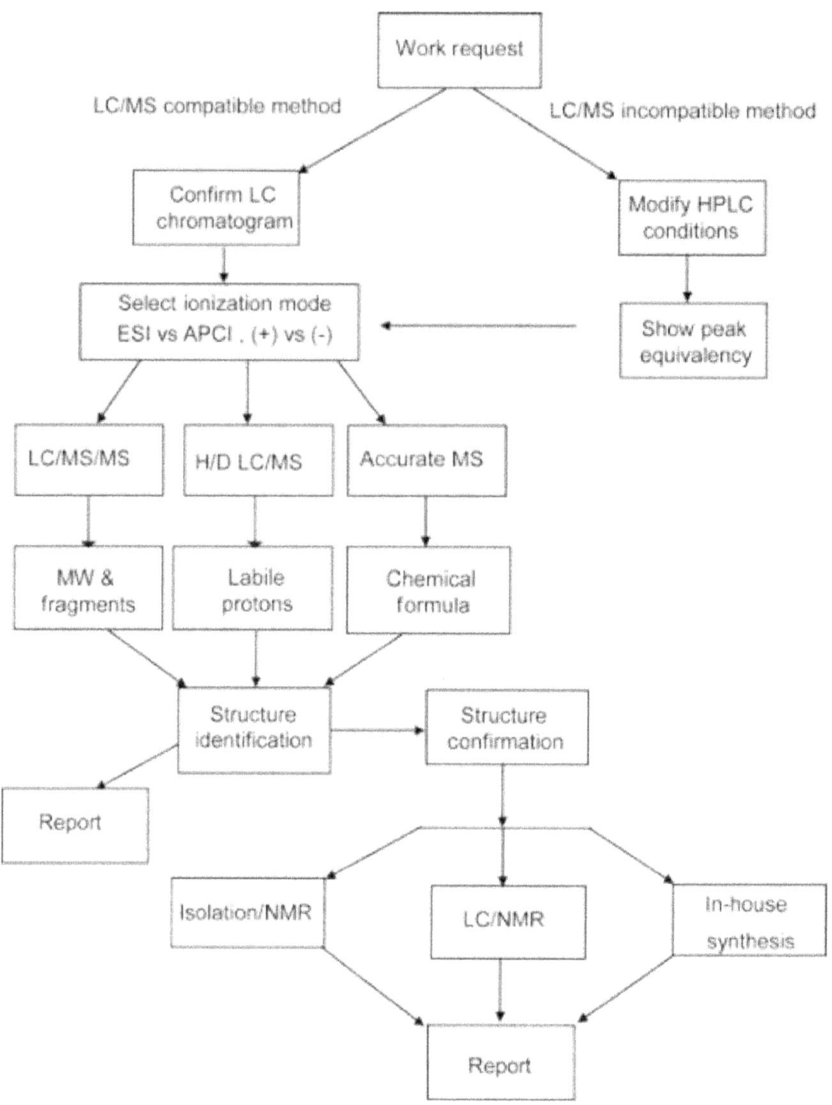

Work request
LC/MS compatible method
LC/MS incompatible method
Confirm LC chromatogram
Modify HPLC conditions
Select ionization mode ESI vs APCI . (+) vs (-)
Show peak equivalency
LC/MS/MS
H/D LC/MS
Accurate MS
MW & fragments
Labile protons
Chemical formula
Structure identification
Structure confirmation
Report
Isolation/NMR
LC/NMR
In-house synthesis
Report

Chapter 12

LC-MS Applications

Mass spectrometry is a very sensitive technique and having good selectivity. In case pharmaceutical bio-analytical samples from clinical trials, it is must to isolate the target analyte (drug) from a sample containing thousands of other different molecules (serum, plasma, urine etc.). Hence, mass spectrometry alone is cannot differentiate compounds by their mass-to-charge ratio (m/z) which is not adequate for practical applications. For example, there are more than 1,500 compounds exists with same molecular mass at around 250 Da. Therefore, an additional separation technique (LC) is needed before presenting the sample to the mass spectrometer. Thus, Liquid chromatography-mass spectrometry (LC-MS) is the combination of two selective techniques (hyphenated technique) which spate the analyte(s) of interest from a complex mixture based on their, physico-chemical properties and MS differentiates analytes based on their mass-to-charge ratio. Due to the dual selectivity nature of LC-MS, it is regarded as powerful analytical tool for biological sample. The LC-MS spectra are appended below (Figure 12.1).

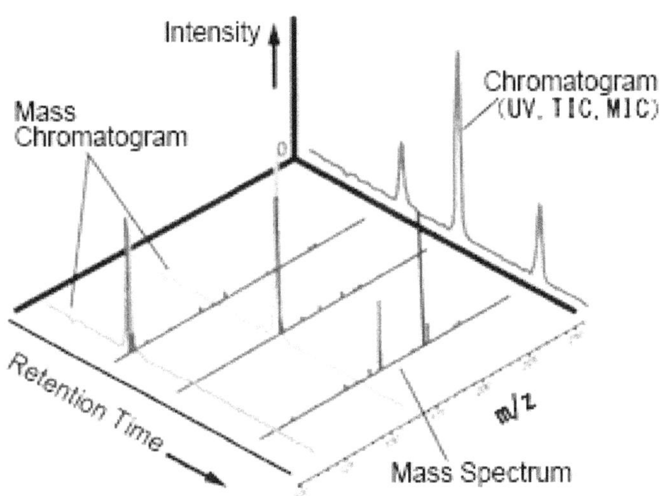

Figure 12.1 LC-MS Spectra.

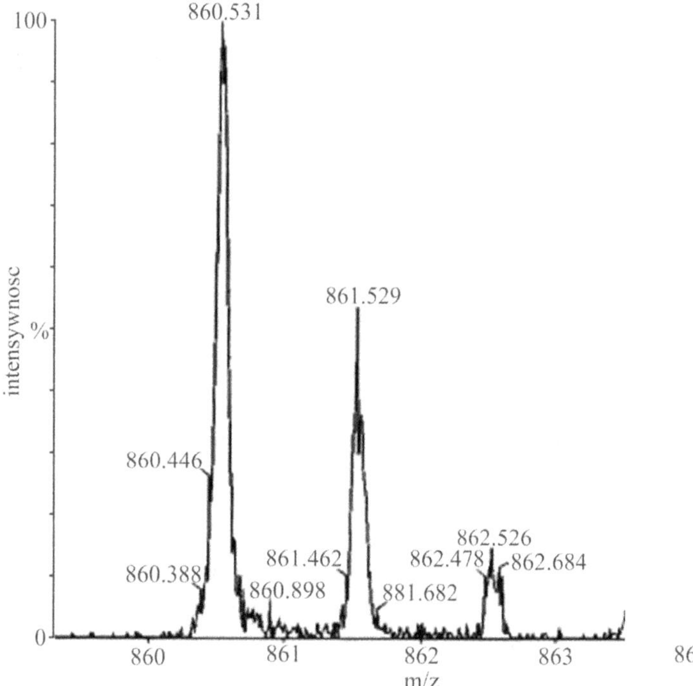

Figure 12.2 Mass Spectra.

Example, the above mas spectrum shows, (Figure 12.2) molecular weights 860.5, 861.5, 862.5. The peak area these peaks are directly proportional to the concentration of the respective ions.

Table 12.1 Advantages and disadvantages of LC-MS

Advantages	Disadvantages
Selectivity: Combining the two separation mechanisms of LC and MS/(MSn) allows the analysis of complex mixtures. Since analytes are separated by their mass-to-charge ratio (*m/z*) the technique allows for the use of isotopically labelled internal standards, which may not separate by LC but can be separated by their mass difference.	Expensive: Mass spectrometers that can couple to LC systems are expensive which are also requires regular servicing is also required, adding to the cost. The environmental conditions in the laboratory need to be well controlled to ensure system stability.
Speed: Since the MS will distinguish Compounds based on mass, the chromatographic method does not have to separate every single component in the sample, so co-elution of non-isobaric analytes is	*Complexicity*: In their own right, both LC and MS can be difficult to optimise. Care must be taken to choose conditions for optimum sensitivity and reproducibility. Sufficient training is also needed to

Table 12.1 contd...

possible. This allows fast LC analysis times and reduced sample preparation, which helps with method development and high throughput sample analysis.	allow analysts to run the systems effectively.
Selectivity: Mass spectrometry is an inherently sensitive technique. Good selectivity also leads to reduced noise, allowing very low levels (fg mL-1) to be detected.	*Limited dyanamic range*: Compared to other quantitative techniques LC-MS has limited range where ranges should not exceed 500-fold concentrations. *Excessive selectivity*: Its due to matrix effect, and very low sensitivity.

Instrumentation

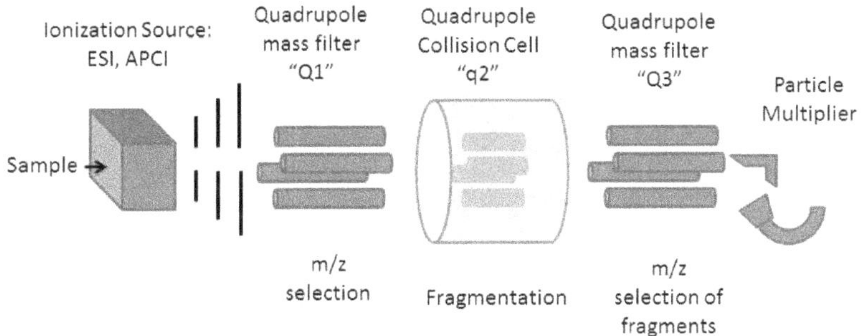

Figure 12.3 Instrumentation.

Ionization source: The direct coupling of LC and MS (LC-MS) has developed into one of the most powerful techniques for trace quantitative analysis. The main breakthrough was solving the problem with the incompatibility of introducing the flow of liquid mobile phase from the LC column into the vaccum required in the mass spectrometer by the use of atmospheric pressure ionisation (API) interfaces. Today, electrospray ionisation (ESI) and atmospheric pressure chemical ionisation (APCI) are the most common API techniques in routine use for quantitation of small molecules by LC-MS. Atmospheric pressure photoionisation (APPI) was developed to increase ionisation efficiencies of non-polar compounds such as polyaromatic hydrocarbons and steroids. The choice of the most appropriate ionisation technique, as well as detection polarity, is based upon analyte polarity and LC operating conditions but many classes of compounds perform well using either technique and sometimes in both ion modes. The selection of ionic source and different mechanism of ionic sources are shown below (Figure 12.4).

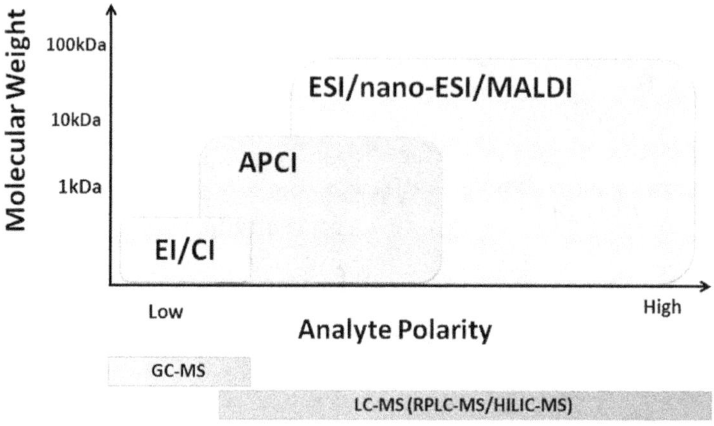

Figure 12.4 Choice of ionization technique based on analyte.

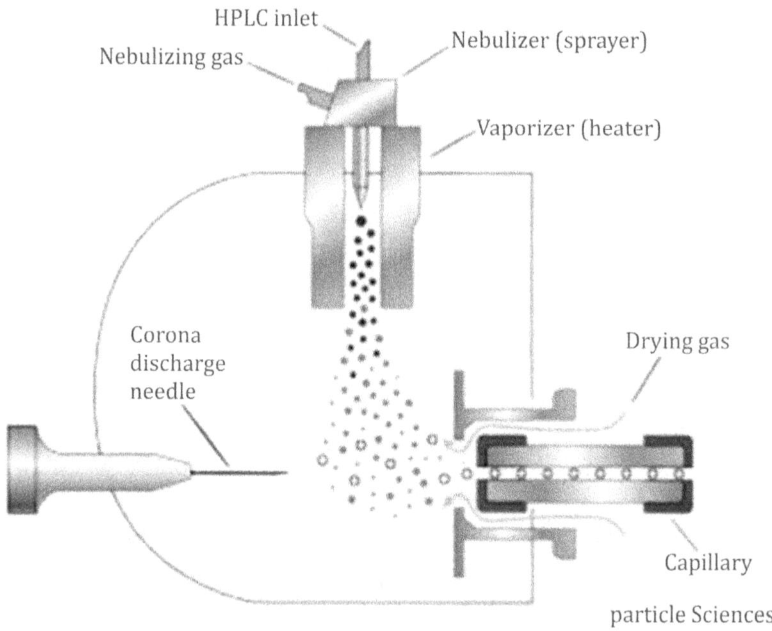

Figure 12.5 APCI ion source in LC-MS/MS.

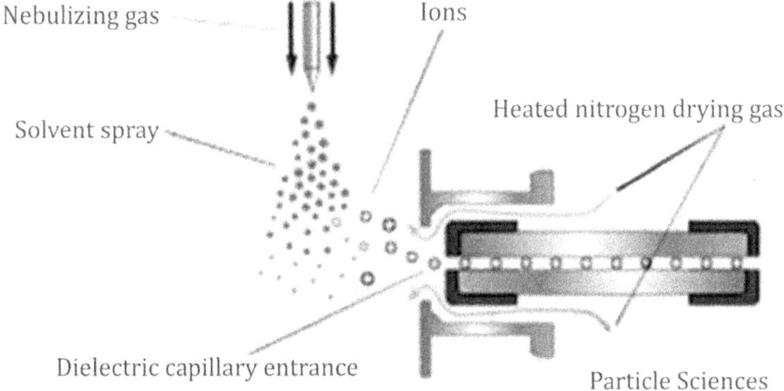

Figure 12.6 Electrospray ion source in LC-MS/MS.

Various stages in LC-MS Method Development

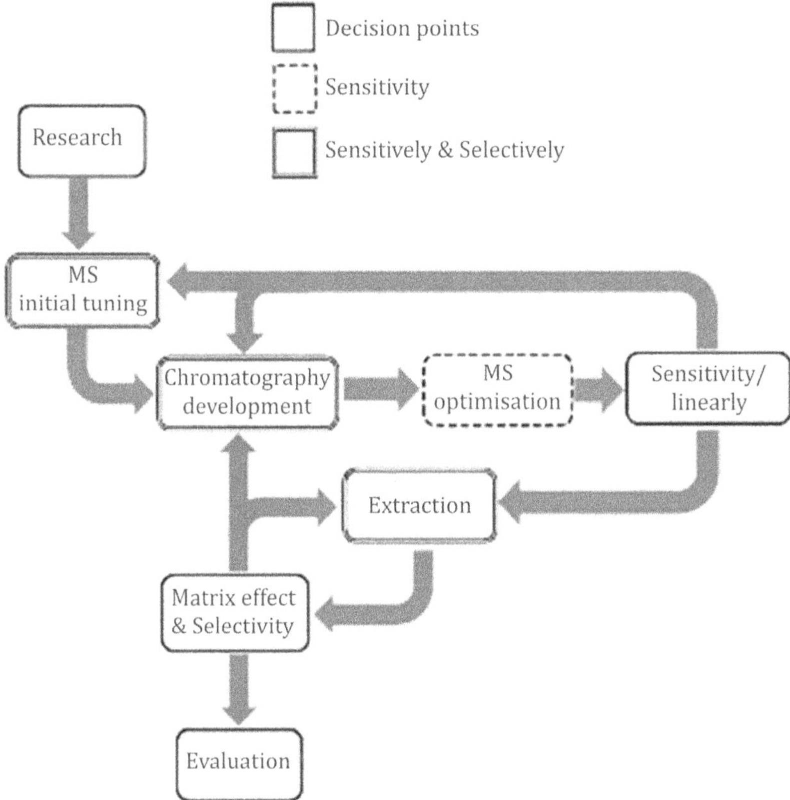

Figure 12.7 Various stages in LC-MS method development.

The most common modes of acquiring LC/MS data are:

- Full scan acquisition resulting in the typical total ion current plot (TIC)
- Selected Ion Monitoring (SIM)
- Selected Reaction Monitoring (SRM) or multiple reaction monitoring (MRM).

Full Can Ananlysis: The total ion current full mass range plot from a PK analysis is a wild place. The MS total ion current plot is a plot much like an HPLC UV trace except for the fact that the mass spectrometer can detect many more components, UV transparent components. The total ion current is a plot of the total ion current in each MS scan plotted as an intensity point.

Selected Ion Monitoring (SIM): In selected ion monitoring the mass spectrometer is set to scan over a very small mass range, typically one mass unit. The narrower the mass range the more specific the SIM assay. The SIM plot is a plot of the ion current resulting from this very small mass range. Only compounds with the selected mass are detected and plotted. The reason for this is because the peaks seen in the SIM plot may only be very minor components in the TIC plot above. The SIM plot is a more specific plot than the full scan TIC plot.

Multiple Reaction Monitoring (MRM) also called Selected Reaction Monitoring (SRM): Multiple reaction monitoring is the method used by the majority of scientists performing mass spectrometric quantitation. MRM delivers a unique fragment ion that can be monitored and quantified in the midst of a very complicated matrix. SRM plots are very simple, usually containing only a single peak. This characteristic makes the MRM plot ideal for sensitive and specific quantitation.

Sample Preparation Technique in LC-MS

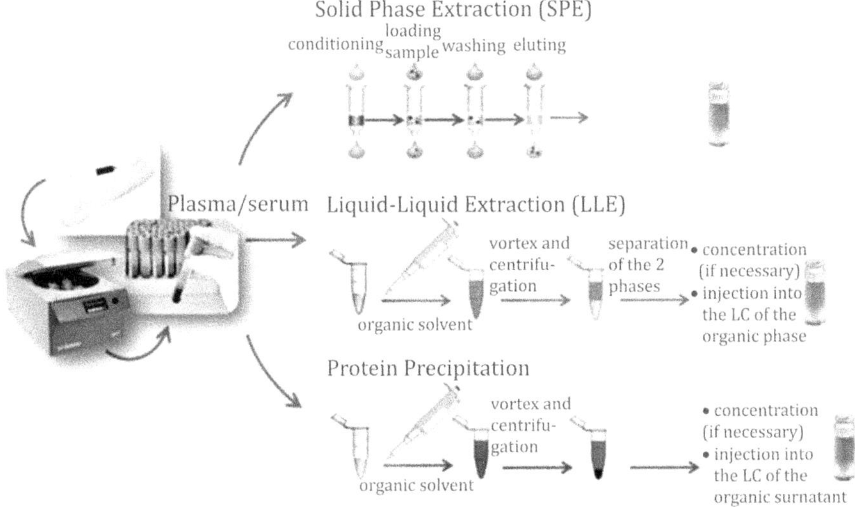

Figure 12.8 Sample preparation technique in LC-MS.

Table 12.2

Protein Precipitation (PP)	Liquid-Liquid extraction (LL)	Solid phase extraction (SPE)
Salting out: Ammonium sulphate is the salt usually used for salting out, because of its high solubility and high ionic strength (which is proportional to the square of the charge on the ion. Neither ion associates much with proteins, which is good since such association usually destabilizes proteins. Solvent Precipitation: When large amounts of a water miscible solvent such as ethanol or acetone are added to a protein solution, proteins	Liquid/liquid extraction is the most common technique used to separate a desired organic product from a biological matrix. The technique works well if your target compound is more soluble in one of two immiscible solvents. The Nernst distribution law states that any neutral species will distribute between two immiscible solvents so that the ratio of the concentration remains constant. $KD = Co/Caq$ Where KD is the distribution constant,	Solid phase extraction is the very popular technique currently available for rapid and selective sample preparation. Many sample preparation methods today rely on solid-phase extractions, an advantage being that SPE is amenable to automation and parallel processing. SPE evolved to be a powerful tool for isolation and concentration of trace analysis in a variety of sample matrices. The most common retention

precipitate out. The conventional wisdom is that this is due to decrease of the dielectric constant, which would make interactions between charged groups on the surface of proteins stronger. Water miscible solvents associates with water much more strongly than do proteins, so that its real effect is to dehydrate protein surfaces, which then associate by van der Waals forces, at least if they are isoelectric or reasonably close to	Co is the concentration of the analyte in the organic phase, and Caq is the concentration of the analyte in the aqueous phase. If KD is very low or the sample volume is high, it becomes nearly impossible to carryout multiple simple extractions in a reasonable volume.	mechanisms in SPE are based on van der Waals forces (—non-polar interactions□), hydrogen bonding, dipoledipole forces (—polar□ interactions) and cation-anion interactions (—ionic□ interactions). It is based on Normal Phase and ion-exchange mechanisms.

Protein Precipitation (PP): In practice, solvent precipitation is usually performed at low temperature. The condition for the protein is at 0°C and the solvent colder, - 20°C in an ice-salt bath, because proteins tend to denature at higher temperatures though if sufficient control can be achieved and your protein is more stable than others, this can be selective and achieve greater purification. Solvent precipitation can be done with polyethylene glycol at concentrations between 5 and 15%. **Demerits:** May increase the back pressure of the HPLC system. Some components of plasma which are soluble in diluting solvent that bound to stationary phase permanently that will affect the column performance

Liquid-liquid extractions (LLE): LLE can separate four different classes of compounds: a. *Organic bases: Any organic amine can be extracted from an organic solvent with a strong acid such as 1M hydrochloric acid; b. Strong acids: Carboxylic acids can be extracted from an organic solvent with a weak base such as 1M sodium bicarbonate; c. Weak acids: Phenols can be extracted from an organic solvent with a strong base such as 1M sodium hydroxide; d. Non-polar compounds stay in the organic layer.*

Solid Phase Extraction (SPE): *There are various stages involved in SPE, they are A)* **Conditioning:** Solvent is passed through the SPE material to wet the bonded functional groups (Use methanol).

B) **Equilibration:** Sorbent is treated with a solution that is similar (in polarity, pH, etc.) to the sample matrix to maximizes retention. (Use the same aqueous solution that the sample is prepared in). C) **Sample Load:** Introduction of the sample so that analytes of interest are extracted onto the sorbent. Must be an aqueous solvent. D) **Washing:** Use the strongest aqueous solution that will not elute the target compounds. Increasing the % organic, increasing or decreasing the pH, changing the ionic strength for increasing clean-up. Dry the cartridge to remove all water. E) **Elution** Use the weakest organic solvent that will remove all of the target analyte. Polar target compounds elute best in polar solvents so in order of polarity try:

methanol>acetonitrile>ethylacetate>acetone>THF. Modify the pH, increase the ionic strength. F) **Solvent exchange:** The organic elution solvent should be evaporated and the sample reconstituted in starting mobile phase.

Merits: Very Selective; Effective with variety of matrix; Concentration effect; High recoveries; High reproducibility.

Demerits: Greater complexity; Lengthy method development; Costly. The various solvent used in SPE Vs intensity signal are shown in the below figure (Figure 12.19).

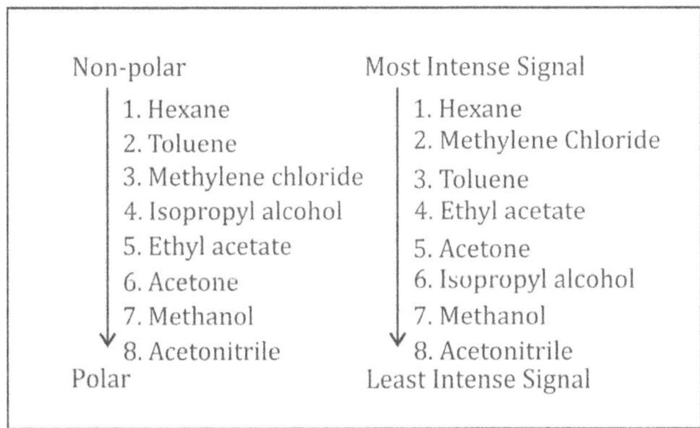

Figure 12.9 Solvent used vs intensity signal.